STUDY OF
CLINICAL COSMETOLOGY-2
A Hands-on Guide

STUDY OF CLINICAL COSMETOLOGY-2

A Hands-on Guide

Sonia Tekchandani MBBS DMLS DDV
Consulting Dermatologist
Tender Skin International
Mumbai, Maharashtra, India

Foreword
Amani Landoulsi

JAYPEE
The Health Sciences Publisher
New Delhi | London | Panama

Jaypee Brothers Medical Publishers (P) Ltd

Headquarters

Jaypee Brothers Medical Publishers (P) Ltd
4838/24, Ansari Road, Daryaganj
New Delhi 110 002, India
Phone: +91-11-43574357
Fax: +91-11-43574314
Email: jaypee@jaypeebrothers.com

Overseas Offices

J.P. Medical Ltd
83 Victoria Street, London
SW1H 0HW (UK)
Phone: +44 20 3170 8910
Fax: +44 (0)20 3008 6180
Email: info@jpmedpub.com

Jaypee-Highlights Medical Publishers Inc
City of Knowledge, Bld. 235, 2nd Floor, Clayton
Panama City, Panama
Phone: +1 507-301-0496
Fax: +1 507-301-0499
Email: cservice@jphmedical.com

Jaypee Brothers Medical Publishers (P) Ltd
17/1-B Babar Road, Block-B, Shaymali
Mohammadpur, Dhaka-1207
Bangladesh
Mobile: +08801912003485
Email: jaypeedhaka@gmail.com

Jaypee Brothers Medical Publishers (P) Ltd
Bhotahity, Kathmandu
Nepal
Phone: +977-9741283608
Email: kathmandu@jaypeebrothers.com

Website: www.jaypeebrothers.com
Website: www.jaypeedigital.com

Inquiries for bulk sales may be solicited at: jaypee@jaypeebrothers.com

Study of Clinical Cosmetology-2

First Edition: **2017**

ISBN: 978-93-86261-90-8

Printed at Sanat Printers

Dedicated to

All my clients and students
who have been my constant source of motivation
to continue my on-going research in the field of
cosmetology and medical esthetics

Foreword

I was introduced to this warm and soft-spoken doctor of Mumbai (India) at an exhibition in Dubai by her very joyful and outgoing husband Deepak, only a couple of years back. Since then we have become very good friends and work associates in Dubai.

It has been a great pleasure for me to write a foreword for Dr Sonia's second book titled, *Study of Clinical Cosmetology-2.*

I have also had the opportunity to read the already published Volume 1 and the transcript of the Volume 2. Both the volumes of this book are an amazing example of how cosmetology as a science of skin beauty can be understood in its absolute simplicity. It entails all topics in extreme detail with its practical application in day-to-day patient interaction. The beauty and wellness industry in India has great potential for growth and work opportunities. I would definitely recommend all the aspiring doctors, skin estheticians and beauty therapists who want to make a career in cosmetology to keep these books as a reference point for their clinical practice.

Dr Sonia is a wonderful human being, a great doctor and a perfectionist in every aspect. The book is so well penned that it makes an easy reading for anyone either from the medical fraternity or other fields.

I am very happy for Sonia and really hope that she keeps sharing her knowledge and continues to write many more books in the future as well.

Amani Landoulsi
PhD Maxillofacial, Plastic and Esthetic Surgery
Associate Professor at the Faculty of Medicine Tunis-Tunisia
Vice President, the Tunisian Society of Esthetic Surgery
Former Asst. Faculty Nantes, Nancy, Grenoble, Strasbourg, France

Preface

This is the second volume of my book—*Study of Clinical Cosmetology* that was published in March 2015 by M/s Jaypee Brothers Medical Publishers (P) Ltd, New Delhi, India. The response and feedback by industry experts, my students and colleagues to the first volume motivated me to put together my second book. This book is a continuation to provide an in-depth understating of the clinical aspects of esthetic medicine. In this volume, I have tried my best to cover procedures best suited for the ever-growing concerns faced by practitioners like pigmentation, scars, stretch marks, fine lines, wrinkles, etc. This book along with its preceding volume would act as a perfect handbook for anybody wanting to introduce the most result oriented and versatile bouquet of services in cosmetology at their esthetic clinic, beauty salon or medi-spa. I have also included advance anti-wrinkle treatments like botulinum toxin and fillers in detail and highly recommend these procedures be performed only by trained medical professionals and under the guidance of senior dermatologist or plastic surgeons. Being a consulting cosmetic-dermatologist for many years now, I have realized that skin is one of the most complex organs of our body and cosmetic procedures can only cure/enhance/improve client concerns to a limited extent. As an esthetician/doctor/counselor, you must understand that you are not only the client's skin consultant but in some capacity a surgeon, a psychologist, an image consultant everything put together and you must also be a very good listener to be able to set their expectations for the desired result correctly. I hope you find this volume informative and use it as a reference guide in your day-to-day practice.

May we continue to add glowing faces to this beautiful world.

Sonia Tekchandani

Acknowledgments

The second volume of the *Study of Clinical Cosmetology* has only been possible because of the amazing response of each one of my readers. A big thank you to all. Thanks to my dear friend and guide, Dr Amani Landoulsi for taking time out and writing a foreword for my book. I would like to extend my utmost gratitude to my entire team of Tender Skin International, Mumbai, India who ensured all the proofreading and constantly met the rigorous deadlines. In addition to, all my mentors, my family and friends I have mentioned in my previous book, I would also like to thank Dr Sumit Agrawal (Consultant Plastic Surgeon—Harleys Cosmetic Clinic), Dr Sanjeev Nelogi (International Expert Trainer—Allergan and Botox), Dr Basem Alhalabi (Plastic and Esthetic Surgeon—Royal Doctors Clinic, Dubai), Dr Ahmad Raza (SSR Plastic Surgery), Dr Jayshree Sharad (CEO Skinfiniti and Vice-President CDSI), Dr Vinay Saraf (Consulting Dermatologist and President—ADC), Dr Rashmikant Shah (Consulting Dermatologist—KRS Derma Care and Secretary—ADC), Dr Uday Khopkar (Consulting Dermatopathologist—Dr Khopkar's Clinic and Scientific Chairman—ADC) and Dr Malvika Kohli (Director—Skin Secrets Clinics).

Contents

1

CHAPTER

Types of Peels

INTRODUCTION

Study of Cosmetology Volume 2 is a compilation and in depth study of skin and its appendages in continuation to Volume 1. It is the study of peeling agents in more detail and understanding patient management in different skin conditions like melasma, ice pick scars, uneven skin tone, etc. A quick recap of the layers of the skin before understanding types of peels and peeling agents in more detail.

LAYERS OF THE SKIN—A QUICK RECAP

Epidermis

The epidermis is completely cellular, meaning it is in a constant cycle of producing new cells while older dead skin cells are pushed to the surface to exfoliate. The epidermis is made up of keratinocytes, lymphocytes, melanocytes, Langerhans cells and Merkel cells. Approximately 80–90% of the cells in the epidermis are keratinocytes, with all others interspersed among them. The layers of the epidermis (Fig. 1.1) are listed below:

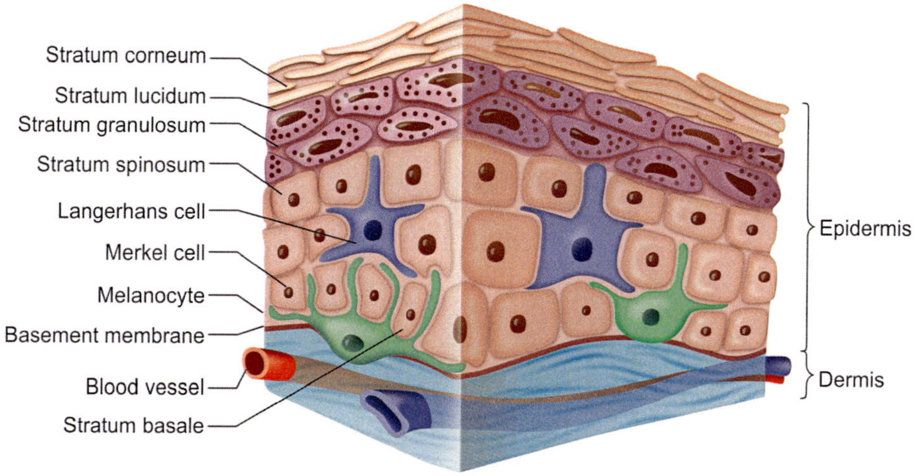

Fig. 1.1: Layers of the epidermis

- Stratum corneum/horny layer
- Stratum lucidum—only present on palms of hands, soles of feet
- Stratum granulosum
- Stratum spinosum
- Stratum germinativum/basal layer.

Dermis

The dermis is a layer of connective tissue, composed mainly of collagen fibers as well as about 5% elastin. The dermis is subdivided into the superficial papillary dermis and the reticular dermis. The papillary dermis is a thin layer of connective tissue fibers, the reticular dermis is thicker and contains collagen and elastin fibers.

Collagen constitutes 75% of dry skin weight, giving the skin volume. Fibroblast cells lie among collagen fibers and are known to synthesize (produce) collagen. Fully mature collagen fibers have a low turnover rate. **Elastin** fibers maintain tension in the skin and provide elasticity (snap back after being stretched). Metabolic turnover for elastin fibers are very slow and only make up about 2–4% of dermal volume. Damage or alterations to the elastin fibers network cause skin to become loose, saggy and wrinkled. **Fibroblasts** are responsible for producing collagen, elastin fibers, and the ground substance of the dermis. Fibroblasts also control the turnover of connective tissue, unfortunately with age they become smaller and less active. The dermis mainly consists of two layers:

- Papillary layer
- Reticular layer (Fig. 1.2).

ACTION AND BENEFITS OF CHEMICAL PEELS

Chemical peeling is used to improve the skin's appearance by applying a chemical solution to the skin, causing the top layers of skin to separate and peel off. The new skin is smoother, less wrinkled and more even in color. Peels can also be used to improve acne. Chemical peels can be performed at different depths, depending on the layer of correction desired. Deeper peels will cause the skin to peel for a longer period of time and provide more improvements in the skin. There are also a variety of acids and peeling agents that can be used alone or together, depending on skin conditions to be treated.

Chemical exfoliation and peels involve using destructive chemical agents to create a controlled wound. All peels (whether they are chemical or laser) create a mild burn. They improve skin by the wound healing process, new tissue is created and damaged tissue is quickly replaced. Chemical peels stimulate the fibroblasts wound healing activity, the proliferation of fibroblast activity increases collagen and elastin. The depth of the wound determines the amount and intensity of healing. The body's response to the burn is what yields the results, a deeper peel will result in more correction.

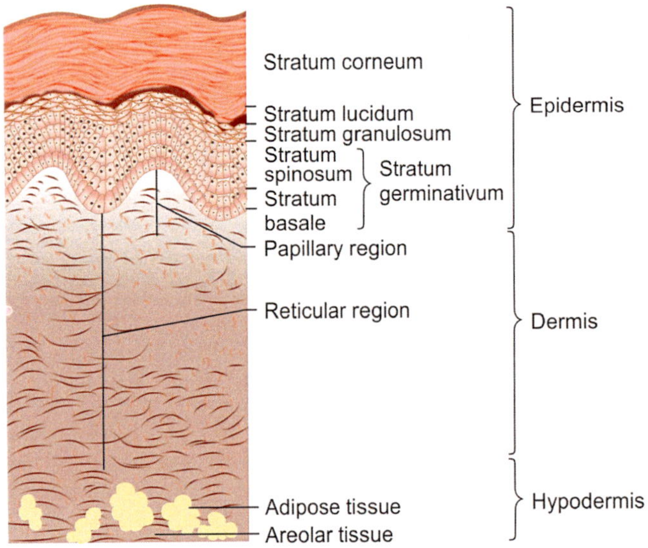

Fig. 1.2: Layers of the skin

The terms exfoliation and chemical peel are often used interchangeably, however superficial peels are technically exfoliation not a true peel. True chemical peels are generally performed under medical supervision, and penetrate into the papillary dermis.

Chemical exfoliation and peels are a way to speed up the natural migration process of skin cells, where the bonds between cells are dissolved and epidermal cells begin to shed more rapidly. The shedding skin cells send signals for more cell division, which in turn forces keratinocytes to the top of the stratum corneum. This process helps treat acne, fade skin discoloration and leave the skin with a fresh new layer of skin on the surface.

DEPTH OF PEELS (FIG. 1.3)

Chemical peeling as we know involves applying a chemical solution to the skin to remove its outer layers. How much skin they remove and how deep they penetrate will depend on the type of peel used, its strength and how long it is left on. There are three types of peel: superficial, medium and deep. These have varying percentages of active ingredients and different pH levels.

Superficial/Light Peels

Superficial or light peels are the gentlest type of peels available and one of the true 'lunchtime' aesthetic procedures. They only remove the top layer of the skin upto the basal layer of the epidermis, and can give your skin and instantly brighter look as well as a smoother, more even texture. They can be used to minimise fine lines and wrinkles, sun damage, mild acne scarring, age spots and dry or flaking skin. They are usually made from alpha hydroxy or beta hydroxy acids, known as AHA's and BHA's and include glycolic acid, lactic acid and salicylic acid. A course of between six to ten treatments is usually recommended to achieve the best results. Superficial peels do not hurt, the patient only feels a slight tingling or stinging sensation, and have virtually no recovery time. The skin can appear to be a little pink afterwards and may get some mild flaking of the skin but this can be disguised with make-up. With a superficial peel the patient is able to return to work or go out straight afterwards (Fig. 1.4A).

Medium Depth Peels

Medium depth peels give more dramatic results than superficial peels. Usually derived from TCA (trichloroacetic acid), they penetrate deeper in to the skin upto the papillary dermis and can be used to treat sun damage, pigmentation and wrinkles. The downside of medium peels is longer recovery and more down time. The patient also feels more discomfort during the treatment than they would with a superficial peel including burning and stinging, which can last for 30 minutes to an hour after treatment. A few days after a medium peel the face can become swollen, pink and itchy following treatment and there is more 'peeling' of the skin then there would be with a superficial peel. The patient may develop patches of brown and white skin on the face during the healing process and in rare cases can get scarring from medium depth peels. Generally recovery takes around a week (Fig. 1.4B).

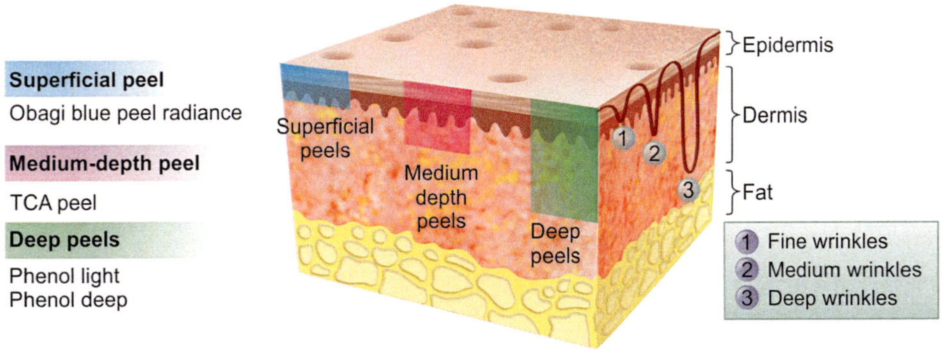

Fig. 1.3: Depth of peels

Deep Peels

Deep peels are the strongest type of chemical peel available and can achieve amazing results for sun damage, scarring and deep lines and wrinkles but the patient must be prepared for a longer downtime after the treatment. They usually use carbolic acid (Phenol peels) or high strength TCA to penetrate the deeper layers upto the reticular dermis of the skin. However, this type of peel is painful and can take a few weeks to months to fully recover. The skin will be very red and feel almost like it is sun burnt after the procedure. Although, you will heal in one to three weeks, the redness can still be visible for months after the treatment but the results of the peel are long lasting. Be warned the patient could feel quite unwell after a phenol peel and may need topical anesthesia during the treatment. It is important to counsel the patient well before the procedure as postprocedure the treated area will be swollen for a couple of days and will then scab. The patient will witness visible peeling and the skin may be quite itchy. For some people it can take up to two weeks before they want to go out in public. The most common problem associated with deep peels is patches of white or bleached looking skin, known as hypopigmentation, which can be permanent. There is also a risk of scarring. Because of the risks associated with Phenol peels it is incredibly important you evaluate the patient's skin type and medical history in detail (Fig. 1.4C).

PEELING AGENTS (FIG. 1.5)

Glycolic Acid

It is the most common peeling agent. It comes in different strengths (30–70%) and different pH levels (levels of acidity) which will determine how deep it penetrates and how much peeling you get. It can be used to treat fine lines and wrinkles, sun damage, improvement of skin texture, skin brightening.

Salicylic Acid

It is unique amongst the hydroxy acids in that it can penetrate deeper into the oil glands causing exfoliation even in the oily areas of the face and scalp, making it ideal for treating acne and oily skin.

Lactic Acid

Occurs naturally in human skin and is also found in milk. It is less irritating than other AHA's and has a natural moisturizing effect on the skin. It is ideal for skin brightening. It can be used to treat pigmentation, dry or dehydrated skin, sensitive skin, rosacea.

Fruit Enzymes

Can also be used as peeling agents. Commonly used fruit enzymes come from fruits, such as papaya, pineapple, pumpkin and cranberry. They are antibacterial, promote cell renewal and can digest sebum and dead cells. They can be used to treat acne, rosacea, dehydrated skin, hyperactive and sensitive skin.

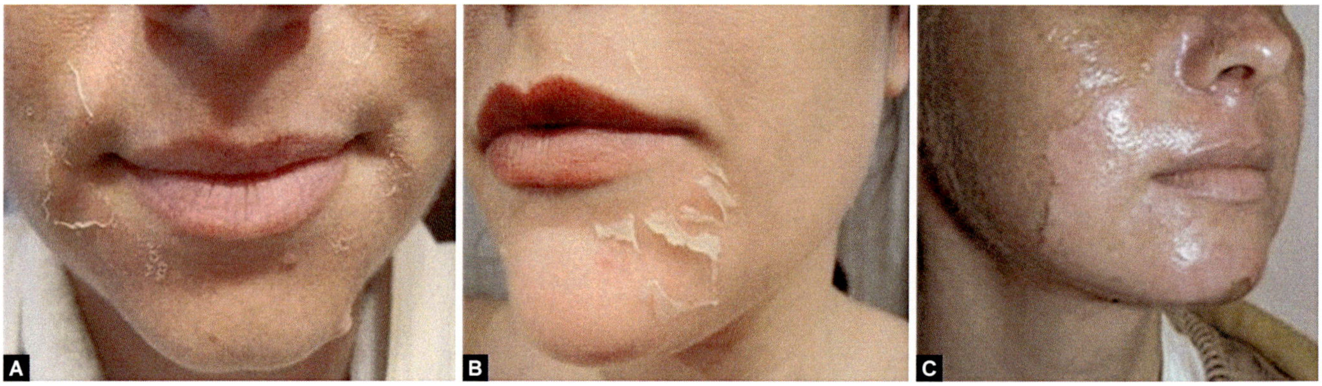

Figs 1.4A to C: (A) Superficial; (B) Medium; (C) Deep peeling

Tartaric Acid

Comes from grapes and is a less irritating alternative to glycolic acid for a milder exfoliation of the skin. It can also help increase hydration. It can be used to treat acne, photo damage, rosacea, superficial pigmentation, eczema.

Malic Acid

Comes from apples and pears and like tartaric acid is a weaker AHA than glycolic acid. It can be used to treat acne, photo damage, rosacea, superficial pigmentation, eczema. Citric acid comes from lemons and oranges and works in the same way as tartaric and malic acids. It can be used to treat acne, photo damage, rosacea, superficial pigmentation, eczema.

Trichloroacetic Acid

Trichloroacetic acid (TCA) is a stronger acid than glycolic. It penetrates deeper into the skin and is usually used for medium depth or deep peels although it can be used at a lower concentration in combination with other acids for a milder peel. It can be used to treat skin tightening, fine lines and wrinkles, acne scars, large pores, hyperpigmentation.

Carbolic Acid

Is found in phenol peels and is the strongest type of peeling agent available. It is used for very deep peels. It can be used to treat deep lines and wrinkles, scarring, severe sun damage.

CHEMICAL PEEL DO'S AND DON'TS

Discourage the Patient to do a Peel Themselves

If done incorrectly chemical peels can cause hyperpigmentation, hypopigmentation and scars. They can find just about anything on the internet these days, however just because they can do something, does not mean they should.

Basic chemical peels	
Very superficial • AHA: Glycolic 20–35%, lactic 50% • BHA: Salicyclic acid 20–30% • TCA: 10–20% • Jessner's: 1–3 coats • Tretinoin and retinol • (Microdermabrasion 2 passes) **Superficial** • AHA: Glycolic 70% • TCA: 20–30% • Jessner's: 4–7 coats • Solid carbon dioxide	Injury of epidermis Minimal downtime All skin types
Advanced chemical peels	
Medium • TCA: 35–40% • TCA: 35% with: • Glycolic: 70% • Jessner's • Solid carbon dioxide **Deep** • TCA ≥50% • Phenol: 88% • Baker–Gordon formula	Injury to dermis Significant downtime Risk of pigmentary changes and other complications

Fig. 1.5: Classification of peels

Abbreviation: AHA, alpha hydroxy acid; BHA, beta hydroxy acid; TCA, trichloroacetic acid

Don't do a Chemical Peel Procedure if

Don't do a chemical peel if the patient is pregnant or on oral or topical retinoids. Don't do medium or deep peels on skin with active acne. Superficial peels are generally recommended when treating skin with acne. One must read the indications and contraindications before suggesting a peel.

Don't Exfoliate

Inform the patient to not do any exfoliating treatments or use exfoliating products until the recommended time, based on the depth of your peel. With medium and deep peels, you should wait at least 3–6 weeks before exfoliating.

Do Brief the Patient to follow Post-treatment Instructions

Use a gentle cleanser and a mild moisturizer. A hydrocortisone cream and antiseptic compresses may also be recommended. White petroleum jelly can be used around areas like the mouth, nose and canthi of eyes to prevent cracking from medium and deep peels. Post-treatment care varies depending on level of peel.

Don't Assist Peeling

Tell the patient don't pick, pull or prematurely remove peeling skin. Removing skin prematurely can cause complications including hyper- and hypopigmentation. Removing skin prematurely will also put the patient at increased risk for infection.

Do Wait for Skin to Peel off on its' Own

Treat the skin almost as if you are trying to keep the peeling skin on.

Don't Hesitate to call if you have Questions or Concerns

If you are unclear about the post-treatment instructions, or are concerned about the reactions contact your doctor.

Do Avoid Cracking and Trauma

Minimize making facial expressions, sleep on your back and avoid letting the shower hit you in the face.

Don't Expose the Skin to Heat or Ultraviolet Rays

Avoid sun exposure and strenuous exercise until peeling is complete.

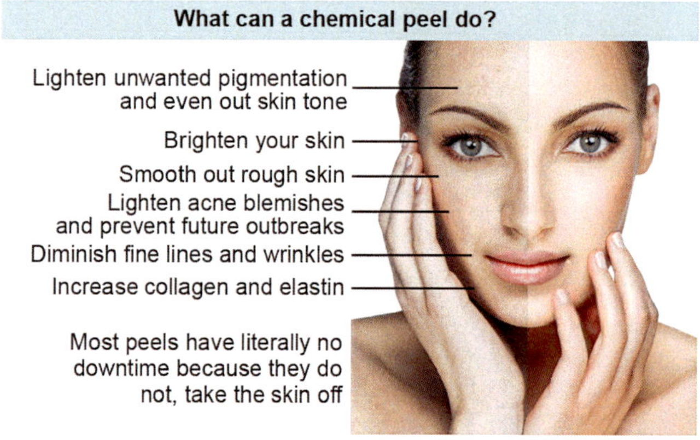

Fig. 1.6: Chemical peel results

Do use a Mineral Powder with SPF or Mild Cosmetic with SPF

Most cosmetics are contraindicated to cosmetic procedures, however mineral makeup can be used immediately after most cosmetic procedures. Mineral makeup has SPF protection and it is not irritating. The cosmetic must not contain talc, it can increase dryness of skin.

Don't Forget to Follow-up

Home care products are recommended and follow-up treatments done to help enhance and maintain results. If you suspect any complications, contact your doctor immediately.

Do have Realistic Expectations

If you are doing a superficial or medium depth peel, please counsel the patient about the results. Do not expect the same results as a deep peel. Even a deep peel cannot replace a facelift, if that's what your patient needs. It is the patient's responsibility to follow post-treatment instructions; noncompliant patients can expect complications (Fig. 1.6).

2
CHAPTER

Advance Peeling Agents

SUPERFICIAL PEELS

Mandelic Acid (Figs 2.1 and 2.2)

- It is an alpha-hydroxy acid derived from bitter almonds, peaches and apricots
- The molecule of mandelic acid is larger and stronger than glycolic acid, hence penetration is slower and less irritating, but still very effective for treating damaged skin
- It is a promising peeling agent for the treatment of all skin types
- It is very superficial peel and effects till stratum corneum
- It is available in the concentration of 20%, 30%, 40% and 50%.

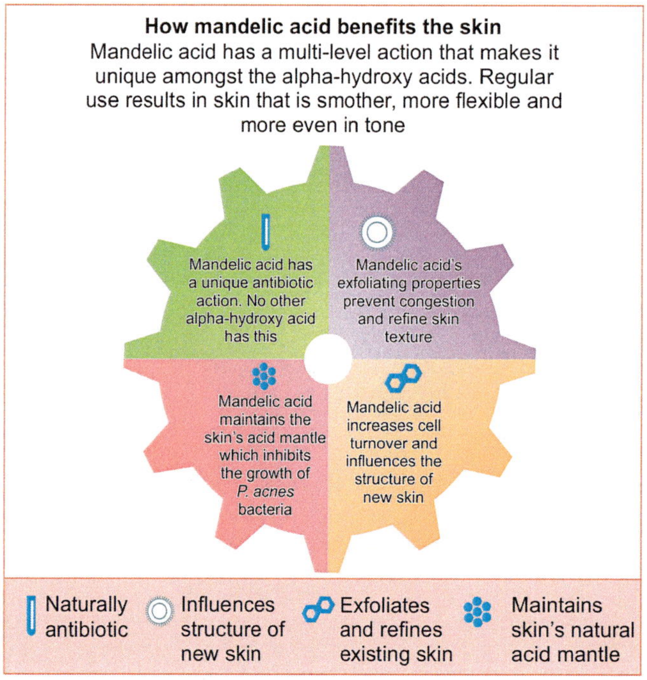

Fig. 2.1: Benefits of mandelic acid

Properties

- It is a great choice for a first time
- It is found to be safer in darker skin types
- It is the least irritating, therefore recommended for sensitive skin
- Breaks down connections between corneocytes of the skin's horny layer leading to its detachment (peeling) of stratum corneum
- Interacts with fibroblast receptors, stimulating the production of collagen in the skin
- Increases moisturization of the skin
- Its anti-bacterial quality also make them good for a people with acne prone skin.

Indications

- Acne
- Stubborn blackheads
- Rosacea
- Pigmentation: Postinflammatory hyperpigmentation (PIH), melasma
- Uneven skin texture
- Anti-aging: Improve the appearance of fine lines
- Skin rejuvenation.

Contraindications

- Active bacterial infection
- Herpes simplex
- Warts
- Open cuts, wounds, inflammation
- Uncooperative patient
- History of photosensitive drugs.

Advantages

- Anti-aging properties are similar to glycolic acid peel, therefore useful in rejuvenating the skin and improving skin texture
- It has antibacterial properties, therefore useful for acne.
- Mandelic acid is stronger than glycolic acid peel, but has large molecular weight which slows penetration making it less irritating
- Mandelic acid does not cause irritation, erythema and burning as compared to glycolic acid peel
- When compared with glycolic acid peels, mandelic acid is less likely to result in crusting, blistering or other adverse effects on the epidermis
- Lack of irritation, burning and erythema are advantages over glycolic acid peel—making it an excellent lunchtime peel.

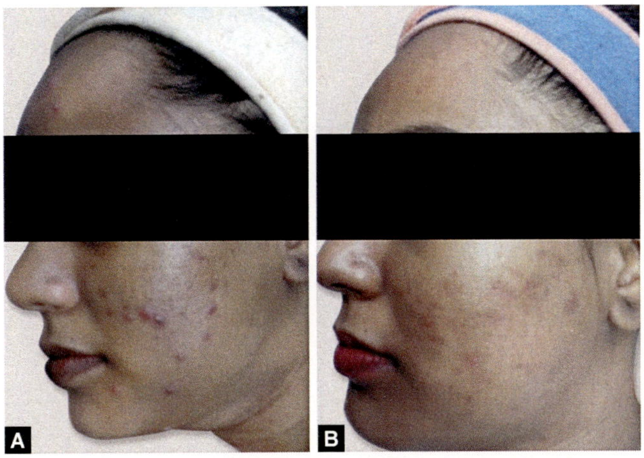

Figs 2.2A and B: Mandelic acid (A) Before and (B) After—28 years/female—5 sessions

Azelaic Acid Peel (Figs 2.3 to 2.5)

- Azelaic acid is a naturally occurring substance found in wheat, rye and barley
- It decreases the production of keratin, which is a natural substance that promotes the growth of acne bacteria
- As a tyrosinase inhibitor, azelaic acid reduces synthesis of melanin.

Properties

- It has anti-inflammatory and antioxidant action
- It is available in 10% and 20% concentration
- It is stronger than retinoids
- It is safe in pregnancy
- It produces antimicrobial effect
- It reduces hyperpigmentation
- It slows the over growth of melanocytes and proliferation of keratinocytes.

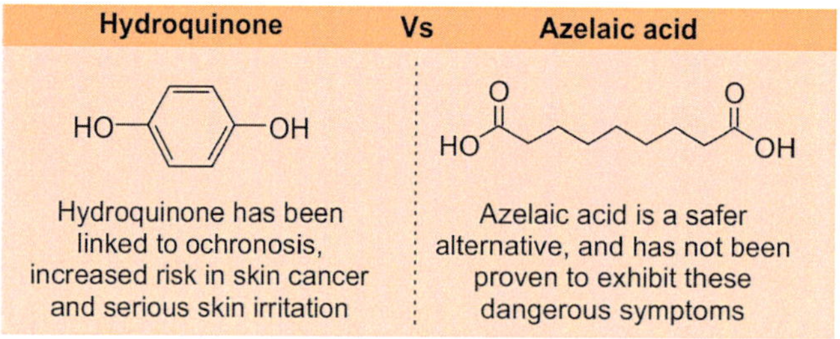

Fig. 2.3: Hydroquinone vs azelaic

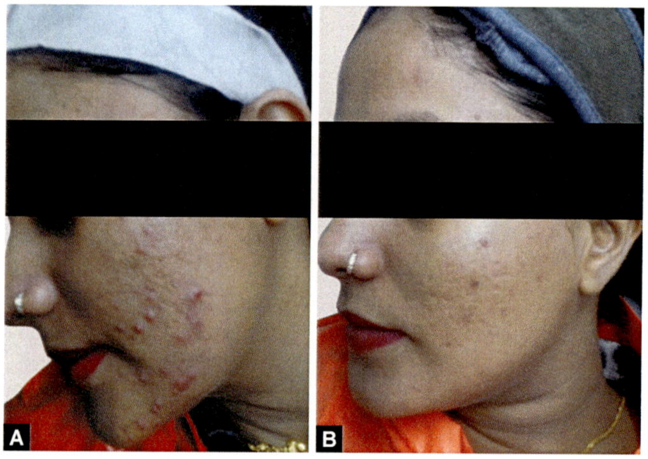

Figs 2.4A and B: Azelaic acid pul (A) Before and (B) after—32 years/female—4 sessions

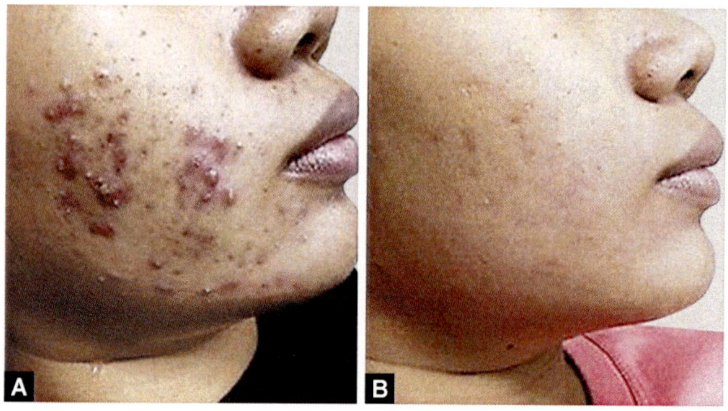

Figs 2.5A and B: Azelaic acid pul (A) Before and (B) after—8 sessions

Indications

- Acne: Comedonal acne and inflammatory acne
- Rosacea
- Perioral dermatitis
- Folliculitis
- Postinflammatory hyperpigmentation
- Actinic lentigines
- Melasma.

Contraindications

- Active bacterial infection
- Herpes simplex
- Warts
- Open cuts, wounds, inflammation
- Uncooperative patient
- History of photosensitive drugs

  Azelaic acid best works for management of acne and postinflammatory hyperpigmentation.

Acne

- It has antibacterial action. It reduces growth of the bacteria in the follicles by inhibiting synthesis of cellular protein bacteria and several oxidoreductive enzymes
- It is anti-inflammatory and reduces postinflammatory hyperpigmentation. It diminishes sebum secretion and improves oily skin
- It has exfoliating properties. It reduces the thickness of stratum corneum and shrinks keratohyaline granules.

Melasma

- It reduces DNA synthesis
- It inhibits tyrosinase activity and melanin synthesis
- It homogenizes color of the skin.

Anti-aging Peel (Figs 2.6 and 2.7)

- It is an alpha, beta, gamma hydroxy peel
- It contains lactobionic acid, gluconolactone and antioxidants which have been suitable for sensitive skin, including rosacea and atopic dermatitis.

  It consists of two phases:

Phase 1

- Alpha-hydroxy acids (glycolic acid, lactic acid, malic acid)—exfoliation
- Beta-hydroxy acids (salicylic acid)—penetration
- Gamma-hydroxy acids (lactobionic acid and gluconolactone)—hydration.

Phase 2

- Antioxidants—Niacinamide, vitamin C + vitamin E, pantothenic acid, vitamin B6.

Properties

- It has a pH-1.80
- It has a larger molecular structure, which causes slower penetration, resulting in reduction of irritation
- Due to their multiple hydroxyl groups, they attract and bind water and have humectant and moisturizing properties
- It is useful in dry and matured skin
- They act as antioxidants hence have good anti-aging properties
- They are not photosensitizing, hence reduce photoaging.

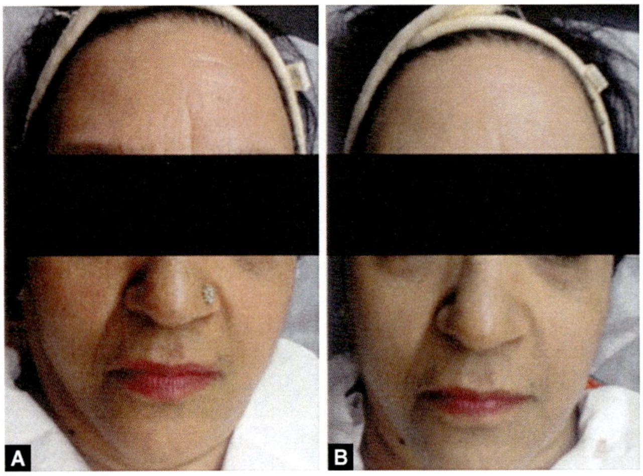

Figs 2.6A and B: Anti-aging peel (A) Before and (B) after—60 years/female—4 sessions

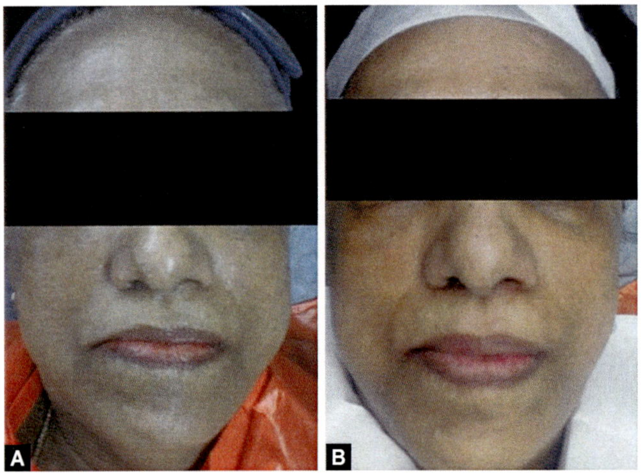

Figs 2.7A and B: Anti-aging peel (A) Before and (B) after—65 years/female—5 sessions

Indications

- Fine lines and wrinkles
- Photo damaged skin
- Solar Lentigines.

Contraindications

- Active bacterial infection
- Herpes simplex
- Warts
- Open cuts, wounds, inflammation
- Uncooperative patient
- History of photosensitive drugs.

Vitamin-C Peel (Figs 2.8 and 2.9)

- It is an alpha-hydroxy acids (AHA) prepared from citrus fruits
- Magnesium ascorbyl phosphate, L-Ascorbic acid, ascorbyl glucosamine and ascorbic acid are various forms of vitamin C

- Advancing age and sun exposure leads to reduction in the capacity of replacing old cells by new healthy cells. This leads to accumulation of dead cells on skin. Vitamin C loosens intercellular substance that holds skin surface cells to each other and sheds damaged skin cells, underneath new cells grow to give fresh look.

Properties

- It is used for all skin types
- It is an effective skin antioxidant
- Inhibits melanin production
- It stabilises oily, acne-prone skin
- It gives a refreshed appearance and a radiant glow
- It improves skin tone.

Sources of vitamin C: Amla (high amount), guava, kakadu plum, orange, lemon, sweet lime, papaya, melon, strawberry, etc.

Anti-oxidant Action

- Fights free radicals that damage the skin and cause photoaging. Improves elasticity
- Fruit acids stimulate cell renewal and cleanse pores
- Helps to repair and heal environmentally damaged skin. It firms and tones the skin
- Can act as a pro-oxidant
- Supports immune system function.

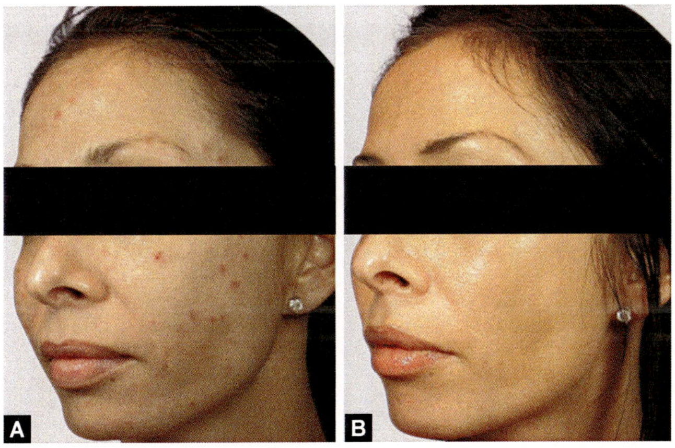

Figs 2.8A and B: Vitamin-C peel (A) Before and (B) after—40 years/female—4 sessions

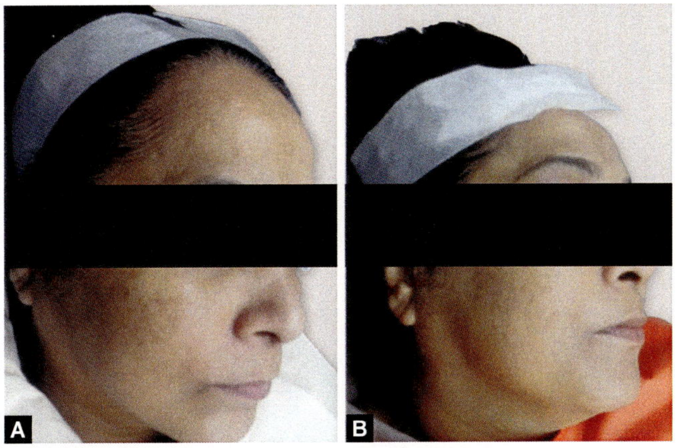

Figs 2.9A and B: Vitamin-C peel (A) Before and (B) after—38 years/female—4 sessions

Anti-aging Action

- Boosts collagen and elastin production
- Smoothens and minimizes fine lines, scars, wrinkles
- Reduces puffiness and helps aging.

Skin Lightening Action

Inhibits tyrosinase activity.

Indications

- Superficial wrinkles on face, neck, arms, upper chest
- Uneven pigmentation
- Enlarged facial pores
- Superficial acne scars
- Acne, oily skin, rosacea
- Post-inflammatory hyperpigmentation.

Contraindications

- Active bacterial infection
- Herpes simplex
- Warts
- Open cuts, wounds, inflammation
- Uncooperative patient
- History of photosensitive drugs.

Benefits

- Improves rough, dry skin
- Exfoliates dead cells
- Slows aging process
- Improves texture of photo damaged skin
- Enhances photo protection
- Normalises and controls oily, acne troubled skin
- Hydrates the skin.

Standard Operating Procedure

- Elevate the client's head by 45 degrees
- Tie Head-band
- Cleanse the face with pre-peel cleanser (to be used according to the skin texture, i.e. oily, normal, dry, etc.)
- Apply petroleum jelly to sensitive areas like outer and inner canthi of eyes, angle of mouth and nose with ear bud
- Explain the procedure to the client in detail
- Peel sensitivity test is to be done (neck, cheek and forehead). This is called 3 point peel sensitivity test
- Apply peel in strokes with a peel brush. As you touch the peel brush on the face start the timer. Strokes should be outward to inwards. Single stroke application is done. Approximate time of application should be 45 seconds and peel to be kept for 3–5 minutes only. These 3 minutes also includes time of application
- Apply cold compresses. If redness or burning is felt before 3 minutes then immediately give cold compresses. Mild itching and burning sensation is experienced which is normal
- Neutralize the peel twice. Neutralization produces a warm sensation due to acid base reaction which is exothermic
- Do not apply neutralizer around eyes and on sensitive skin
- Apply cold compress twice
- Apply face mask (hydrating/whitening) for 15 minutes
- Remove the mask and apply sunscreen according to skin type.

Precautions: While doing the peel if there is unbearable burning, stinging, redness or frosting immediately apply cold compress and if still persists then remove the peel.

Post-peeling Care

- Can wash with plain water after 2 hours
- Soap can be applied after 12 hours
- There will be mild redness for 1–2 hours
- Avoid direct sunlight
- Apply sunscreen 20 minutes before sun exposure
- Avoid swimming and excess sweating for 3–4 days
- No facial, bleach, threading, waxing, plucking for 7 days before and after the peel
- Avoid make-up for 12 hours
- Do not use medicated creams 2 days before and after peel
- Do not pick! Picking delays healing and causes scarring
- Use sunscreens and moisturisers according to skin type.

Protocol

- Interval between 2 peels is 15 days
- Peel should be done 3–4 days before any social commitment
- Minimum 8–10 sessions are required for best results
- Maintenance sessions are required every month.

Side Effects

- Itching and redness which subsides in a week
- Persistent erythema in rare cases.

Note

In Anti-aging peel phase 2 is applied after neutralization.
In vitamin C peel no neutralization is required.

MEDIUM DEPTH PEELS

Yellow Peel (Figs 2.10 and 2.11)

Yellow peel is the latest medium depth chemical peel, which can promote elimination of epidermis at different depths, and it can also be tailored to the type of skin.

- This peeling uses the exfoliant action of retinol in high concentrations together with the action of four substances, (Niacinamide, vitamin C + vitamin E, pantothenic acid, vitamin B6) which block the synthesis of melanin by preventing the transfer of melanin from melanocytes to keratinocytes.

It contains three phases:

- *Phase I:* Contains—Niacinamide, vitamin E, Pantothenic acid, vitamin B6 (pH 6.7)
- *Phase II:* Contains—vitamin C (pH 2.33)
- *Phase III:* Contains—Retinol cream (pH 1.1).

Indications

- Melasma
- Benign hyperchromic lesions of the epidermis
- Superficial wrinkles.

Contraindications

- Active bacterial infection
- Herpes simplex
- Warts
- Open cuts, wounds, inflammation

- Uncooperative patient
- History of photosensitive drugs.

To prepare the stratum corneum for a perfect and uniform penetration of the Yellow Peel first do 2–3 sessions of alpha-beta-hydroxy peel, followed by a session of yellow peel.

Yellow peel should be used in a thin and continuous layer all over the face, or only in the area that needs treatment. The peel should be left on the skin for a continuous period of 12 hours and then removed with water.

Normally, this treatment can be repeated after 3 weeks, depending on the type of skin being treated or as recommended.

Procedure

- Elevate the client's head by 45 degrees
- Tie head-band
- Cleanse the face with prepeel cleanser (to be used according to the skin texture, i.e. oily, normal, dry, etc.)
- Apply petroleum jelly to sensitive areas like outer and inner canthi of eyes, angle of mouth and nose with ear bud
- Explain the procedure to the client in detail
- Apply phase I in strokes with a peel brush. Strokes should be outward to inwards. Single stroke application is done
- Keep the peel on till it dries completely. It takes approximately 10 minutes
- Then apply phase II over it in the same manner as phase I (Single coat only). Let this phase also dry completely
- Lastly, apply phase 3, i.e. retinol cream on it.
- There is yellowish tint immediately after the procedure
- Apply sunscreen. There is dryness for almost one week after the procedure

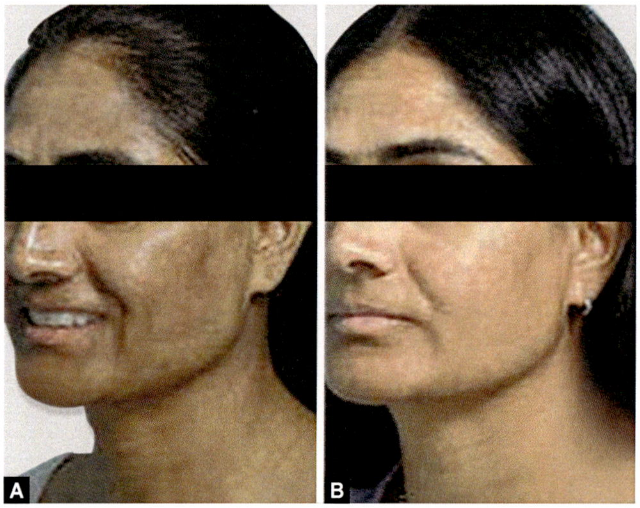

Figs 2.10A and B: Yellow peel (A) Before and (B) after—36 years/female/—5 sessions

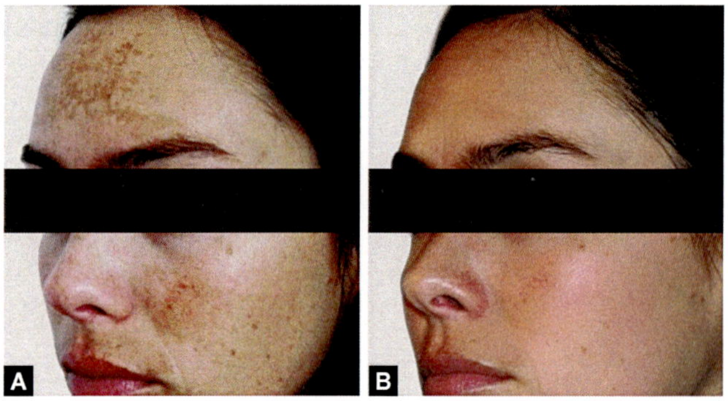

Figs 2.11A and B: Yellow peel (A) Before and (B) after—28 years/female/—5 sessions

- Moisturize liberally
- Mild peeling may be experienced after 2–3 days which settles within a week.

Retinol (Vitamin A) Peel (Figs 2.12 to 2.14)

Introduction

Retinol (vitamin A) peel is suitable for all skin types and will gently remove dead skin cells and promote a healthier looking skin. Face, chest and back can be treated with retinol peel.

There is no heat or unpleasant sensation with the application of Retinol (vitamin A) peel. Retinol (vitamin A) peel can be carried out alone or in conjunction with a microdermabrasion to maximize results.

Properties

- Retinol (vitamin A) peel is suitable for all skin types
- Helps in collagen production, which plums wrinkles and adds youthful appearance.
- It can be used for all age groups (15 years and above).

Indications

- Resistant-pigmentation
- Photopigmentation
- Acne and sequelae of acne
- Skin aging and photo-aging
- Wrinkles
- Loss of skin elasticity and strength
- Disruption of skin' natural moisture balance
- Hyperkeratosis.

Contraindication

- Use of retinol increases the probability of severe skin reaction to treatment
- Atopic skin, eczema, seborrheic dermatitis, etc.—indicate skin hypersensitivity (reactivity)
- Viral infections—under the influence of retinol and acids, can cause reactivation of herpes in patients with a history of herpes
- Warts—can cause further viral shedding from a wart
- Photosensitivity—high skin sensitivity to solar or other types of UV radiation
- Compatibility with pharmaceutical products—those who have taken oral retinoids should wait at least 3–6 months before getting a retinol peel
- Liver diseases, including previous hepatitis infections
- Pregnancy or planning pregnancy within a year, and lactation, as retinoids are embryotoxic.

Procedure

- Elevate the client's head by 45 degrees
- Tie head-band
- Cleanse the face with prepeel cleanser (to be used according to the skin texture, i.e. oily, normal, dry, etc.)
- Apply petroleum jelly to sensitive areas like outer and inner canthi of eyes, angle of mouth and nose with ear bud
- Explain the procedure to the client in detail
- Take 5–10 g of 10% Retinol mask in a bowl
- Apply uniformly on skin including upper and lower eyelids
- The areas of lashes and eyebrows should be avoided. The peel can be performed even on sensitive areas, which is one of the advantages of the retinol peel. It is not recommended to apply the mask to the eyelids if it contains depigmentating components
- The mask sets and becomes firm in 10–25 minutes. Then it is removed
- Skin is treated with a special sunscreen.

The main benefit of the mask is that it forms an occlusive film on skin and stimulates uniform collagen production. The standard retinol peel includes 4 procedures. The interval between the first and the second one is 2 weeks, between the others—1 month. In the future, this kind of peel can be performed for prophylactic purposes as a supportive treatment at intervals of 3 months.

Post-peel Care

When a retinol peel treatment is over, a recovery period begins which requires a special skin care regimen. The use of cosmetic products containing retinoids and AHA is prohibited within two weeks after the treatment. Other cosmetic procedures and procedures that use chemicals, like hair dyeing or hair perms, are not recommended.

Any swelling, irritations, and pain that might appear should be treated with anti-inflammatory and regenerating agents, for instance, with a special gel consisting of borage oil, shea butter, copper peptides, panthenol, extracts of rosebay, liquorice, and horse chestnut. This gel has a soothing effect and helps skin recover faster to its normal state.

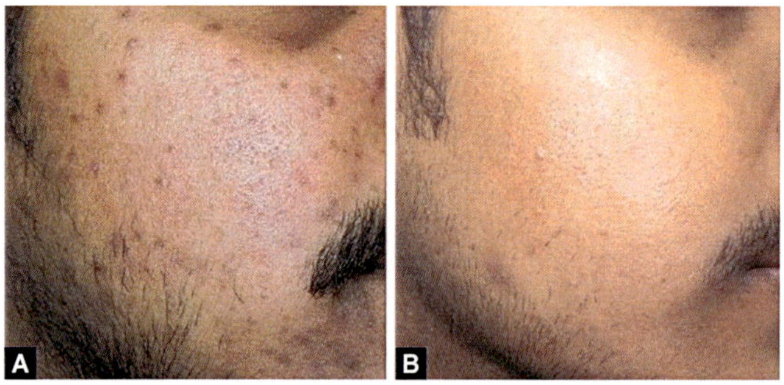

Figs 2.12A and B: Retinal (Vitamin A) peel (A) Before and (B) after—23 years/male—4 sessions

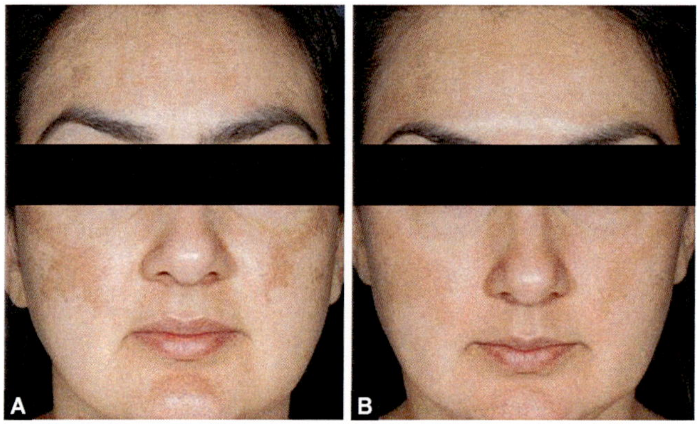

Figs 2.13A and B: Retinal (Vitamin A) peel (A) Before and (B) after—30 years/female—4 sessions

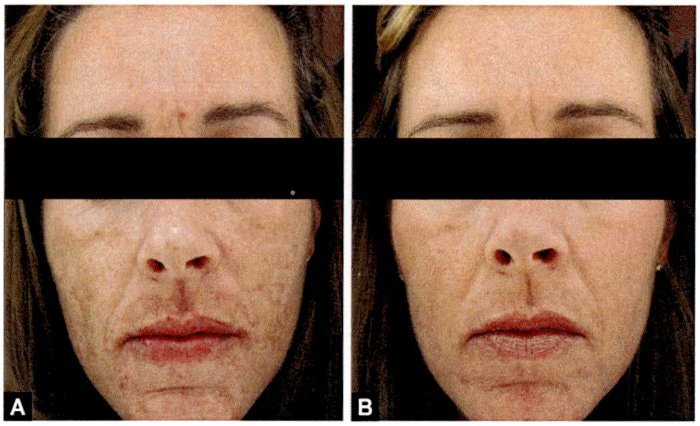

Figs 2.14A and B: Retinal (Vitamin A) peel (A) Before and (B) after—37 years/female—4 sessions

Facial cleansers that contain no hard surfactants can be used on the second day after the peel procedure. Facial cleansers and skin care products should be fat-free, i.e. water-based.

Active skin exfoliation starts in 3–4 days. In order to speed up the process, it is recommended to use a mask rich in lactic acid.

Possible Complications of Retinol Peels

- One of the common side effects of this peel treatment is flaking skin
- Flaking skin becomes darker, which leads to a common side effect as darkening of some skin areas. Things go back to normal when the flaking is over
- Swelling might also occur as a local inflammatory response to external stimuli. People with thin skin (usually on the neck and around the eyes) are most prone to this complication. Swelling normally occurs in 1 to 3 days after the peel which subsides in a week
- Please remember that after the peel skin is highly sensitive to external stimuli, like low and high temperatures, mechanical action, and sunlight (UV component). In some cases, this complication may develop further resulting in hypersensitivity that might last up to 1 year
- There is a high risk of getting an infection during the treatment as the peel considerably reduces immune response. The most common infections, which disturb patients after a peel treatment, are herpes and strepto-staphylococcal pyoderma. The former is treated with antiherpetic agents (acyclovir), the latter with antibiotic drugs and ointments.

Jessner's Peel (Figs 2.15 and 2.16)

- It is a medium depth chemical peel, a combination of alpha- beta-hydroxy acids, i.e. lactic acid and salicylic acid, along with a phenol derivative, i.e. resorcinol
- It can be used alone or in combination with TCA to increase the depth of the peel
- Modified Jessner's peel eliminates resorcinol and includes citric acid, reducing the side effects and decreasing toxicity, while increasing its efficacy.

Action

These molecules act in synergy. Resorcinol is a good peeling agent resulting in renewed stratum corneum and increased density of glycosaminoglycans. Salicylic acid is a lipophilic agent with keratolytic and anti-inflammatory properties.

Storage

It has a shelf life of 2 years. Stored in dark amber colored bottle with a tight cap.

Indications

- Acne
- Sun damaged skin, patchy pigmentation
- Superficial scars
- Dilated pores
- Fine wrinkles.

Contraindications

- Allergy to resorcinol
- Allergy to salicylates
- Pregnancy and lactation
- Active infection
- Acne excoriee or obsessive picker.

Procedure

- Cleanse the required part with a cleanser
- Peel sensitivity test is done

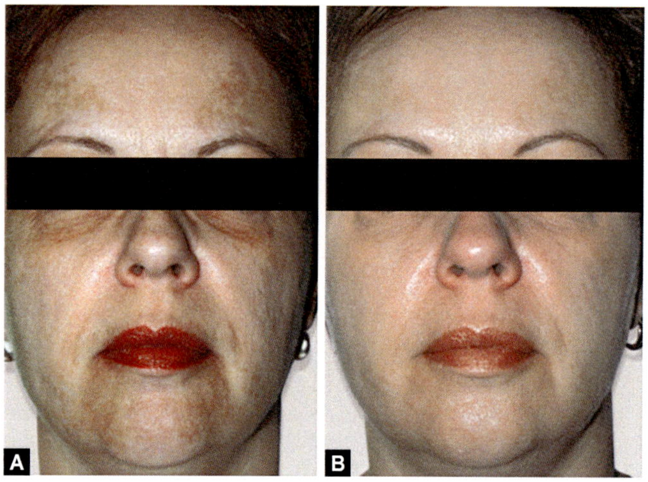

Figs 2.15A and B: Jessner's peel (A) Before and (B) after—46 years/female—6 sessions

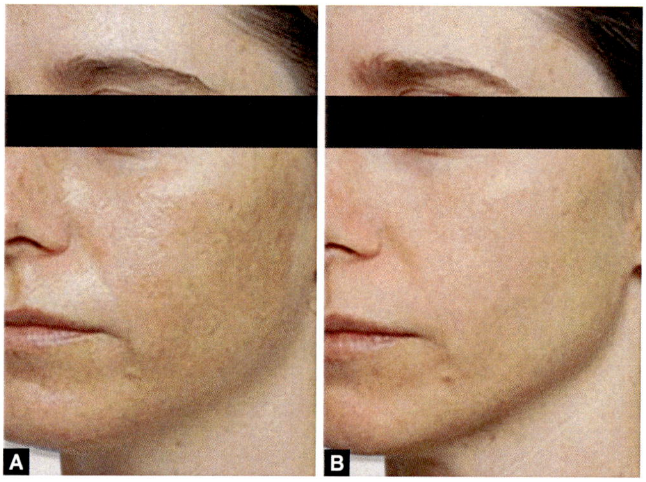

Figs 2.16A and B: Jessner's peel (A) Before and (B) after—38 years/female—5 sessions

- Apply the peel
- Apply 1–2 coats depending on the severity of the pigments. For skin types 4, 5, 6 do not exceed more than 2 coats
- Allow the skin to dry completely between the coats (approx 4–5 minutes)
- No neutralization is required. Cold compression can be given
- Slight erythema with a little frosting is seen in some areas. Mild to moderate amount of burning and stinging lasting for about 15–30 minutes is experienced by the patient. Peeling and exfoliation is seen over the next 2–4 days
- Apply sunscreen according to the skin type. For dry, flaky skin a moisturizer is recommended.

Jessner's peel is a safe peel giving rise to a lot of peeling. It causes a lot of burning, stinging and exfoliation. Useful for acne, photo-ageing and pigmentation.

Phytic Acid (Figs 2.17 and 2.18)

- It is a superficial to medium depth peel
- Phytic acid is an alpha-hydroxy acid with a large molecular weight
- It is composed of three alpha-hydroxy acids with Phytic acid, i.e. glycolic acid, lactic acid and mandelic acid
- It is characterised by high anti-oxidant activity.

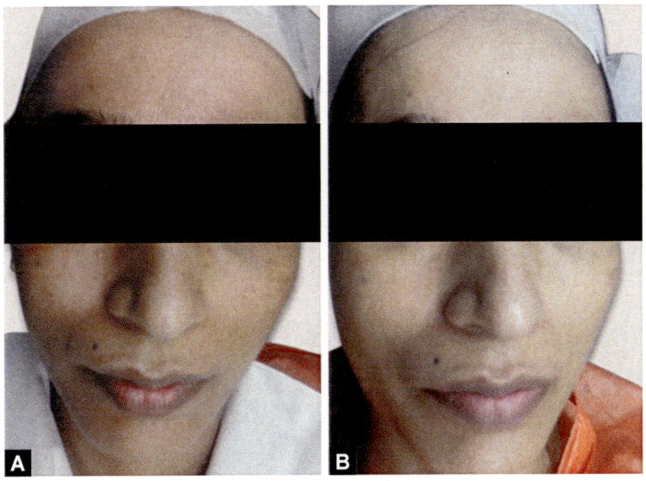

Figs 2.17A and B: Phytic acid (A) Before and (B) after—32 years/female—6 sessions

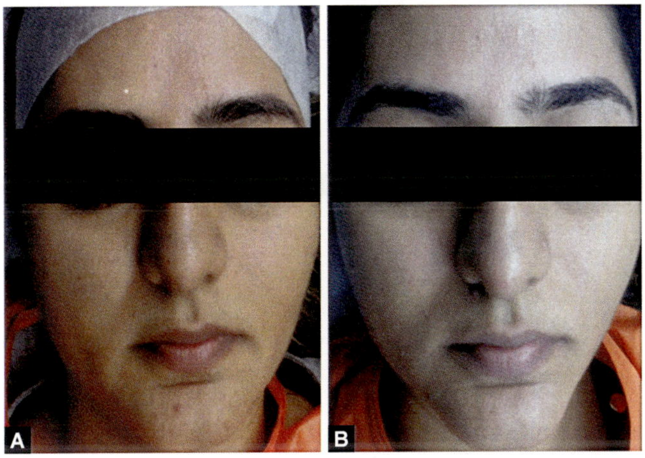

Figs 2.18A and B: Phytic acid (A) Before and (B) after—27 years/female—5 sessions

Properties

- The 3 alpha-hydroxy acids have different rates of penetration in the epidermis. The phytic acid is a large inositol hexaphosphoric acid which fights and neutralizes free radicals, and promotes cell regeneration. No frosting should appear. Frosting occurs in case retinol or other exfoliating agents have been used
- It works best for residual lesions of acne with early erythematous or pigmented scars of grade1 or 2
- Glycolic acid works on regeneration
- Mandelic acid has antibacterial and anti-inflammatory properties
- Lactic acid acts as a hydrant and rejuvenating base
- This is a slow-release, mild superficial peel that is safe for all skin types
- It is also useful for sensitive skin
- It also has strong antioxidant properties
- It is found naturally in cereals such as rice and wheat bran.

Procedure

- Elevate the client's head by 45 degrees
- Tie head-band

- Cleanse the face with pre-peel cleanser (to be used according to the skin texture, i.e. oily, normal, dry, etc)
- Apply petroleum jelly to sensitive areas like outer and inner canthi of eyes, angle of mouth and nose with ear bud
- Always do peel sensitivity test
- Apply 1 ml of phytic acid in strokes with a peel brush. Strokes should be outward to inwards. Single stroke application is done
- Mild itching and burning sensation is experienced which is normal
- Does not require neutralization or cold compresses
- After 5 minutes apply thin layer of anti-inflammatory cream/gel and cling film on the face and remove cling film after 15 minutes
- Left over products can be penetrated into the skin
- Lastly, apply sunscreen according to the skin type.

Precautions: While doing peel if there is unbearable burning, stinging, redness or frosting immediately neutralize the peel with cold compresses.

Advantages: It does not require neutralization. It is a slow, superficial peel for those who do not want a visible flaking of the skin. It can be used safely in all skin types. It evens out the complexion and has a marked lightening effect. It can be repeated once in two weeks to achieve the maximum results.

Disadvantages: Since its a superficial to medium depth peel, its useful only for mild epidermal conditions like superficial hyperpigmentation, smoothening the skin. Requires multiple applications for effect.

Post-peel Care for Medium Depth Peels

- Wash with plain water after 12 hours
- Soap can be applied after 24 hours
- There will be mild redness for 1–2 hours
- Avoid direct sunlight
- Apply sunscreen 20 minutes before sun exposure
- Avoid swimming and sweating for 3–4 days
- No facial, bleach, threading, waxing, plucking for 7 days before and after the peel
- Do not use medicated creams 2 days before and after peel
- Do not pick! Picking delays healing and causes scarring
- Moisturize liberally.

Complications of Medium Depth Peels

- Persistent erythema
- Bacterial infection
- Hyperpigmentation
- Hypopigmentation
- Scarring
- Milia
- Acneiform eruptions
- Demarcation lines
- Reactivation of herpes
- Contact dermatitis
- Hypertrophy/Keloids.

Protocol for Medium Depth Peels

- Interval between 2 peels is 21days
- Peel should be done at least 15 days before any social commitment
- Minimum 4–5 sessions are required for best results
- Maintenance sessions are required every 3 months

DEEP PEELS (FIG. 2.19)

Phenol Plus Peel (Body Peel)

- Phenol plus peel is made of products intended to maintain the thickness of the stratum corneum and dermoepidermal cell renewal
- It has a hydroalcoholic base
- It contains formulation which contains some or most of these solvents like phenol, trichloroacetic acid, retinoic acid and a mixture of hydroxy acids (glycolic acid, ascorbic acid, salicylic acid and mandelic acid) with phytic acids
- As the name suggests, phenol plus peel can be done on any area of the body except face and some other sensitive areas
- It penetrates till the reticular layer of the skin.

Properties

- Non-buffered hydroalcoholic solution pH—0.5
- Painless procedure (no analgesics are required)
- Deep acting peel
- The depth of the peel depends on the number of coats applied
- There is no risk of hypopigmentation or hyperpigmentation.

Indications

- Post-inflammatory hyperpigmentation
- Melasma
- Resistant pigmentation
- Amyloidosis
- Dermal pigmentation
- Superficial wrinkles.

Contraindication

- Pregnancy and lactation
- Active infection
- Sensitive skin
- Uncooperative client
- Recent cuts or wound on concerned area.

Procedure

- Cleanse the required area
- Apply the peel, 1-2 coats depending on the severity of the pigments. In patients with skin types 1, 2 and 3, 2 to 3 coats are recommended and skin type 4, 5 and 6, do not exceed more than 1 coat in the first session and do not apply more than 2 coats in later sessions

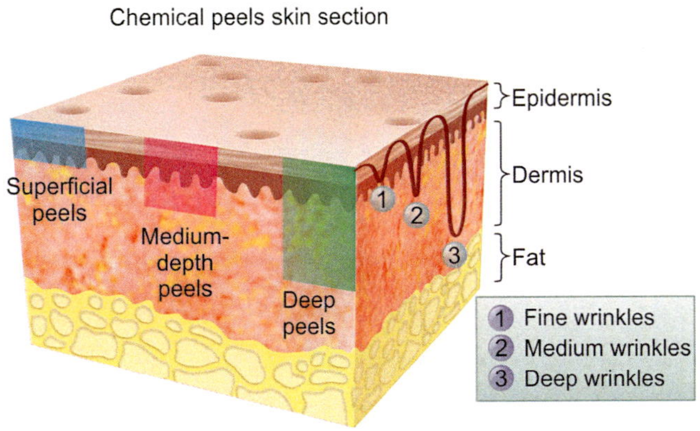

Fig. 2.19: Deep peel targeted layer

- Allow skin to dry completely between the two coats
- A maximum application of 5 mL product is recommended per session
- Depending upon the brand and composition you are using, you may leave on the peel or neutralize it
- Apply retinol cream
- Lastly apply sunscreen
- Peeling and scaling of skin start after 3–4 days of treatment and continue for 7–10 days
- Results are seen in 7–10 days. There is renewed and bright complexion. Homogenous skin color and texture.

Trichloroacetic Acid (Figs 2.20 to 2.25)

Trichloroacetic acid (TCA) is formulated on a hydro-glycerinated base. It is a versatile peeling agent and is useful as a superficial, medium and deep peel as per concentration (Tabel 2.1).

Properties

- The depth of the peel correlates with concentration
- In dark skins, 10–15% is safe, but concentration beyond 25% has high risk of pigmentary changes
- It is safer to combine two peeling agents in lower concentration sequentially rather than increase concentration
- Renews epidermis and increases fibroblastic activity, which synthesizes the different macromolecules of the extracellular matrix
- Reorganizes collagen and elastin fibers, improving physiological and mechanical qualities of the skin
- Chemical reconstruction of skin scars (CROSS) technique is useful for post-acne ice pick scars.

Actions

It causes coagulation of skin proteins leading to frosting. Precipitation of proteins leads to necrosis and destruction of epidermis. Coagulation is followed by inflammation and activation of mechanisms of wound repair. This leads to epithelialization with replacement of smoother skin with an even tone. There is collagen remodeling with production of new collagen. It is self-neutralizing and hence not absorbed in systemic circulation.

TABLE 2.1: TCA peel effects as per concentration

Depth	*Skin layer*	*Effects*
Very superficial	Intraepidermal	Erythema
Superficial	Basal layer	Frosting points
Medium depth	Grenz zone	Frosting clouds
Deep	Papillary dermis	Even pink color with frosting

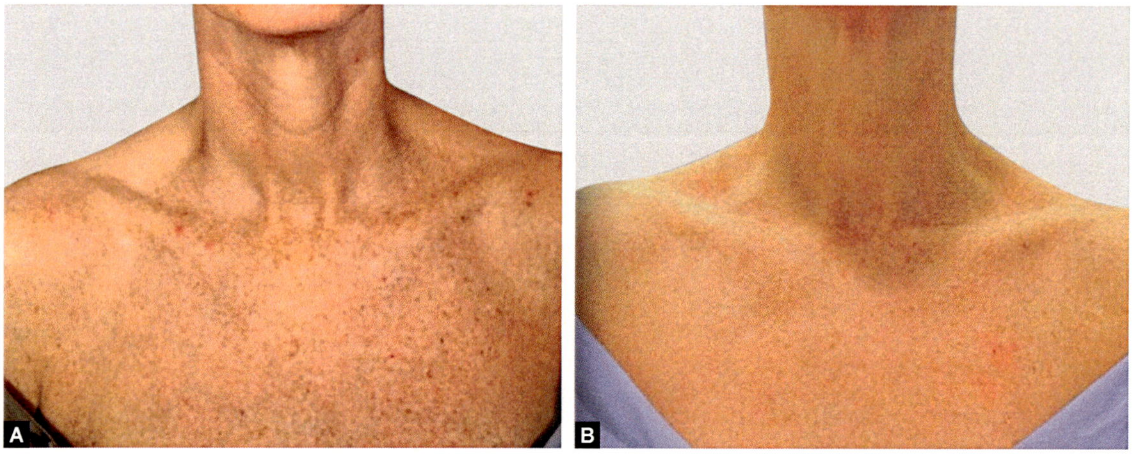

Figs 2.20A and B: Trichloroacetic acid (A) Before and (B) after—42 years/female—5 sessions

Cross Technique (Fig. 2.26)

A technique consisting of the application of higher TCA 40–65% concentrations by pressing hard on the entire depressed area of atrophic acne scars. This technique is called chemical reconstruction of skin scars (CROSS).

Performed for fibrotic, superficial as well as ice pick scars, deep rolling and boxcar scars. Excellent improvement in 3–5 sittings conducted at monthly intervals.

Repeated CROSS application destroys the atrophic pit with restructuring and thickening of dermal collagen.

Best results are seen for fibrotic, ice pick, boxcar scars and dilated pores.

CROSS method with micromesotherapy in same session targets improvement in most scars of grade 2–3.

Indications

- Photoaging
- Melasma

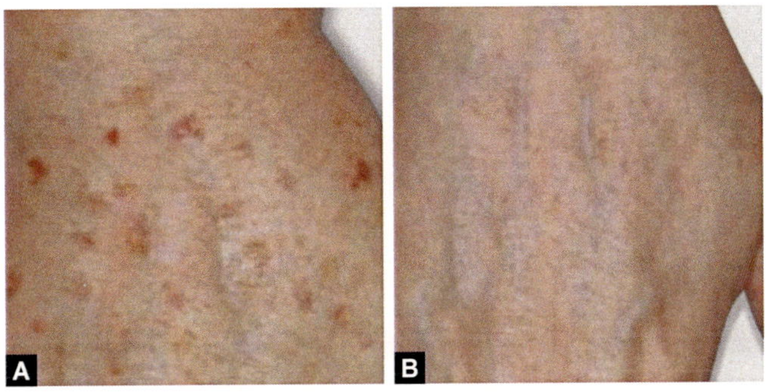

Figs 2.21A and B: Trichloroacetic acid (A) Before and (B) after—32 years/female—4 sessions

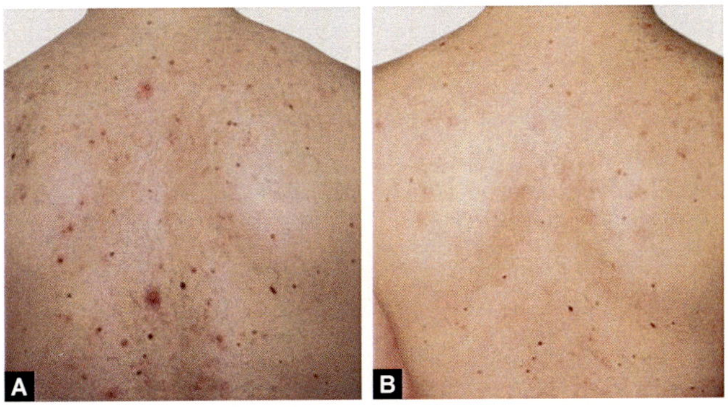

Figs 2.22A and B: Trichloroacetic acid (A) Before and (B) after—35 years/male—5 sessions

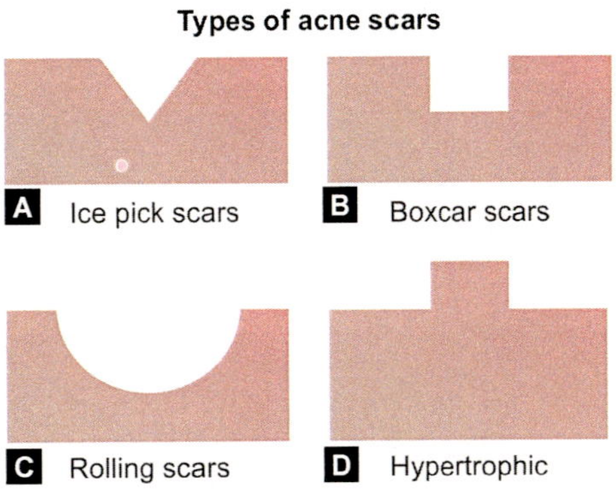

Figs 2.23A to D: Types of scars

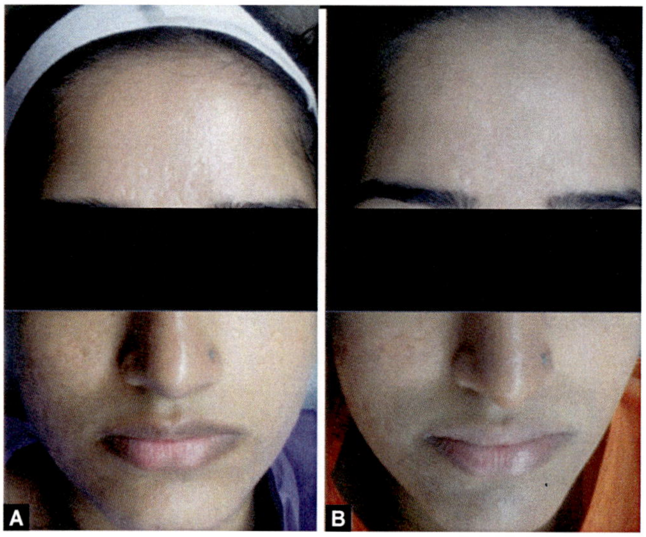

Figs 2.24A and B: Trichloroacetic acid (A) Before and (B) after—28 years/female—4 sessions

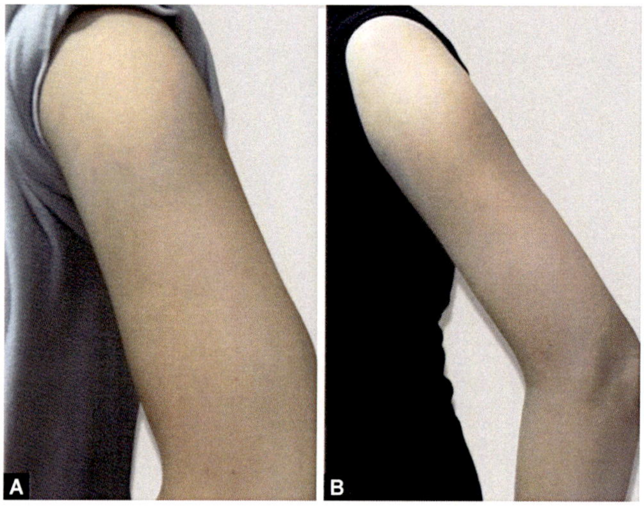

Figs 2.25A and B: Trichloroacetic acid (A) Before and (B) after—25 years/female—5 sessions

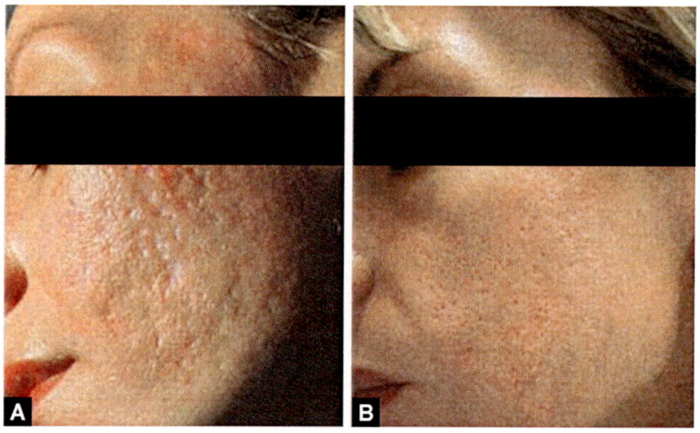

Figs 2.26A and B: TCA cross technique (A) Before and (B) after—38 years/female—5 sessions

- Post-inflammatory hyperpigmentation
- Acne scars
- Actinic and seborrheic keratosis
- Lentigines
- Freckles.

Contraindications

- Active bacterial infection
- Herpes simplex
- Warts
- Open cuts, wounds, inflammation
- Uncooperative patient
- History of photosensitive drugs.

Procedure

- TCA 10–15% is used for superficial peels (up to stratum corneum)
- TCA 25% used as medium peels (up to basal layer of epidermis)
- TCA 10–15% can be used on face. Beyond TCA 15%, it is to be used on the body.
  - Cleanse the required area with pre-peel cleanser (to be used according to the skin type, i.e. oily, normal, dry, etc.)
  - Always do a peel sensitivity test
  - Explain the procedure to the client in detail
  - Take informed consent and before and after photo of the client
  - Apply TCA peel in strokes with a peel brush. Single stroke application is done. If redness or intolerable burning is felt, then immediately apply cold compresses
  - Mild itching and burning sensation is experienced which is normal
  - The end point of the peel is white frosting with minimal or no erythema
  - Peel will flake lightly and heal in 4–7 days. In cases of deeper peels, second coat is required which takes 7–10 days to heal
  - Apply sunscreen according to the skin type.

Post-peel Care for Deep Peels

- Wash with water after 12 hours of treatment
- Avoid soap or facewash 24–48 hours after treatment
- Client is strictly advised to avoid direct sun exposure or remain indoors
- Moisturization is a must after this treatment
- Patient will feel tightness of the skin after a peel
- Sunscreen and moisturizers are used till desquamation subsides
- In superficial peels little or no peeling occurs with flaking and scaling at few places
- Darkening of skin returns to normal in 2–7 days. If crusting occurs, topical anti-bacterial ointment is used to prevent bacterial infection
- Peels are repeated every 3 weeks, till improvement which occurs after 4–6 peels.

Protocol for Deep Peels

- Interval between 2 peels is 3–4 weeks
- Minimum 4–5 sessions are required for best results
- Maintenance sessions are required every 3 months.

Complications of Deep Peels

- Persistent erythema
- Bacterial infection
- Hyperpigmentation

- Hypopigmentation
- Scarring
- Milia
- Acneiform eruptions
- Demarcation lines
- Reactivation of herpes
- Contact dermatitis
- Hypertrophic scars/Keloids.

Common Side Effects of Deep Peels

- There will be itching and redness that subsides after one week
- Peeling of skin
- Dryness of skin.

SPECIAL PEELS

Melasma Mask (Figs 2.27 to 2.29)

Description: Deep exfoliating peel done monthly to even the layers of the skin, promote exfoliation of the skin's surface layers, favor cell renewal, improve the texture of the skin, and reduce the signs of aging. It can be done for brides and grooms.

Kit Contains

- *Degreasing solution:* Alcohol, acetone
- *Pre-peel solution:* Salicylic acid
- *Mask:* Kojic acid, Azelaic acid, citric acid, ascorbic acid, lactic acid, arbutin, glycyrrhetinic acid, phytic acid, salicylic acid, tocopheryl acetate
- *Regenerating gel:* Hyaluronic acid, hydrolyzed collagen, tocopheryl acetate, ascorbic acid, aloe. Propylene glycol, chamomile, calendula
- *Maintenance cream:* Kojic acid, azelaic acid, citric acid, ascorbic acid, lactic acid, arbutin, glycyrrhetinic acid, phytic acid, salicylic acid, tocopheryl acetate.

Indications

- Melasma
- Resistant pigmentation
- Thick and rough skin
- Uneven skin texture
- Fine lines
- Wrinkles
- Skin glow.

Contraindications

- Active acne
- Active skin infection
- Sensitive skin.

Procedure

- Explain the procedure to the client in detail. Take informed consent and before and after photo of the client
- Apply degreasing solution to prepare the skin for treatment. This solution eliminates impurities and excess sebum from the epidermis and is able to lower the pH of the skin, allowing a greater penetration of the active ingredients in the mask
- Apply pre-peeling solution which helps eliminate dead skin cells from the epidermis
- Apply mask over the face, to form a thick layer on the concern area. Apply half of the contents of the jar and leave half for a second application 21–30 days after initial treatment

- Keep the mask on the face from 8 hours to 12 hours depending on skin type. Timings will vary for each individual patient. The patient may experience different sensations, such as slight itching or feeling of warmth or tingling feeling
- The patient will go home with the mask applied
- After 8–12 hours remove the mask with water. There may be erythema or a sensation of heat may be felt
- *Day 1:* After removing the mask, the patient should immediately apply the regenerating gel on the entire treated area and repeat the operation several times throughout the day

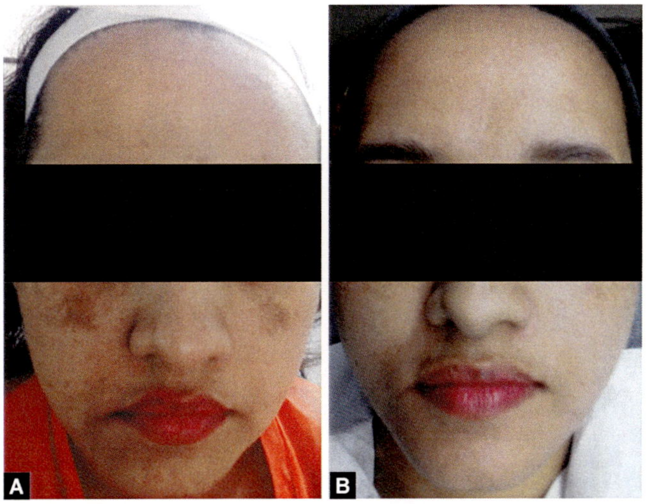

Figs 2.27A and B: Melasma mask (A) Before and (B) after—28 year/female—2 sessions

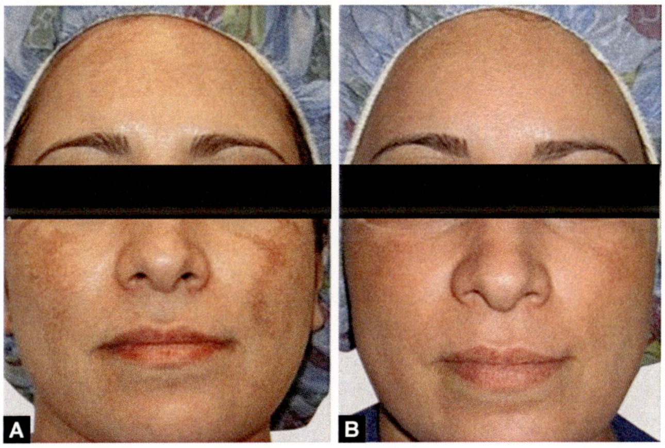

Figs 2.28A and B: Melasma mask (A) Before and (B) after—36 years/female—2 sessions

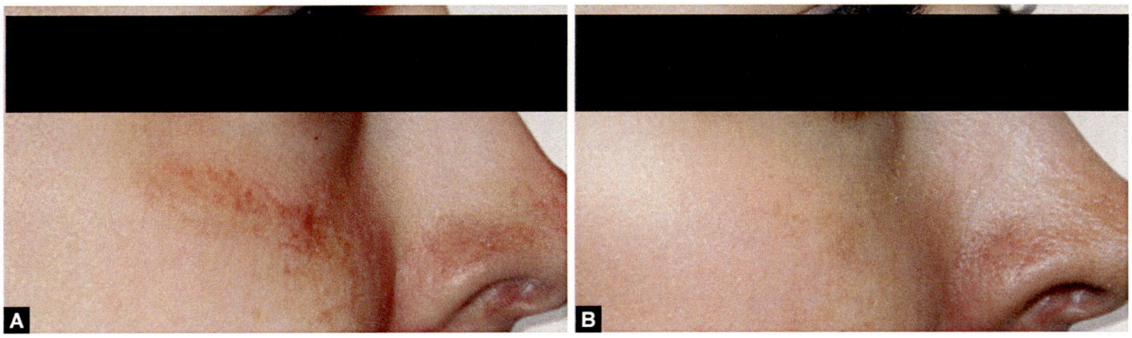

Figs 2.29A and B: Melasma mask (A) Before and (B) after—30 years/female—2 sessions

- *Day 2 to the next 4 weeks:* Apply maintenance cream 2 times a day. After 15 minutes apply regenerating gel on top.
- *From 5th week to 12th week:* Apply maintenance cream once a day
- *From the 13th week to 1 year:* Apply maintenance cream on concern areas
- It is recommended to use a sunscreen daily with a high protection
- Mild peeling may be experienced after 2–3 days which settles within a week.

Note: Kit can be used for 2 sessions for same client or single session for 2 different clients.
Depending on type of skin the mask can be left for 8–12 hours.
Skin type 1 and 2–8 hours
Skin type 3 and 4–10 hours
Skin type 5 and 6–12 hours.

Precautions

While doing peel if there is unbearable burning, stinging, redness or frosting immediately give cold compresses.

Repetition

Interval between 2 peels is 30 days.

Advantages

- Only 2 sessions 1 month apart are required in a year
- Maintenance session is required once a year only.

Black Acetic Acid Peel (Figs 2.30 to 2.33)

The black acetic acid is a natural organic acid. Black peel is made from the fermentation of black rice. It contains large amount of organic materials, minerals and high concentration of essential amino acids.

Contains

- Black acetic acid
- Salicylic acid
- Jasmonic acid
- Potassium iodide.

Properties

- It is an antioxidant and anti-bacterial
- It has skin lightening effect similar to arbutin which is a tyrosinase inhibitor
- Helps to improve various skin problems like acne, skin aging and pigmentary problems
- Potassium iodide is an anti-fungal agent which works well on livedo vasculitis. Helps in faster wound recovery
- Acne spot cream has biosulfur in addition to above which is used as post-treatment home care. It has a ph of 2.7
- It has anti-cancer properties in vivo on rats and in vitro on human cancer cells
- It is easy and safe non-ablative peel.

Indications

- Acne vulgaris grade IV
- Resistant acne
- Adult acne resistant to isotretinoin and relapse post-isotretinoin
- Patients with polycystic ovarian disease (PCOD) who cannot take OC pills
- Acne with post-inflammatory hyperpigmentation and scars.

Contraindications

- Patients on isotretinoin
- Pregnant and lactating females

- Active secondary infection
- Active dermatosis like psoriasis and eczema.

Procedure

- Cleanse the face with the cleanser
- Do comedone extraction if needed

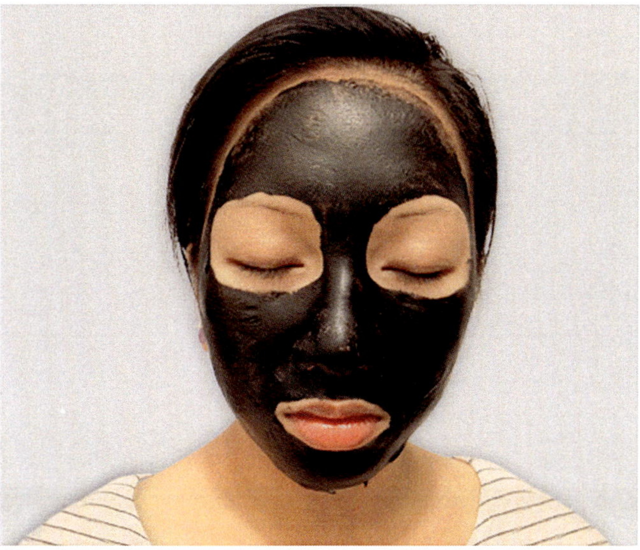

Fig. 2.30: Black acetic acid peel

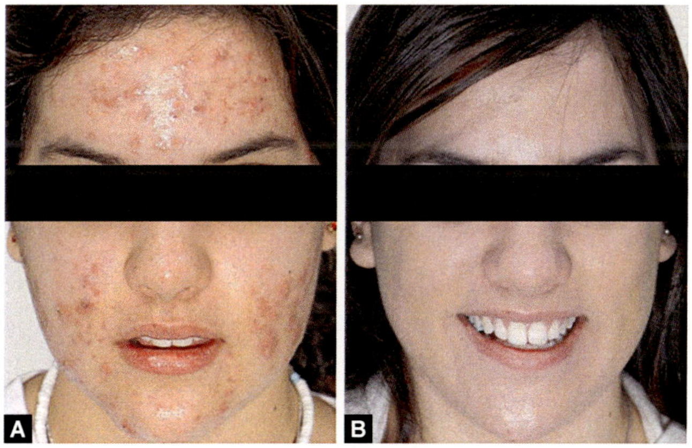

Figs 2.31A and B: Black acetic acid peel (A) Before and (B) after—26 years/female—4 sessions

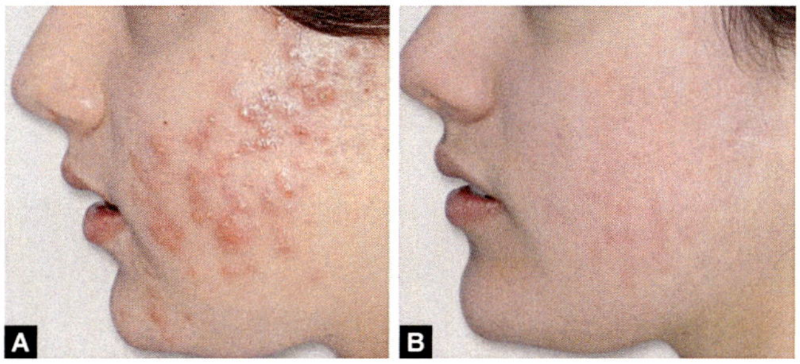

Figs 2.32A and B: Black acetic acid peel (A) Before and (B) after—22 years/female—4 sessions

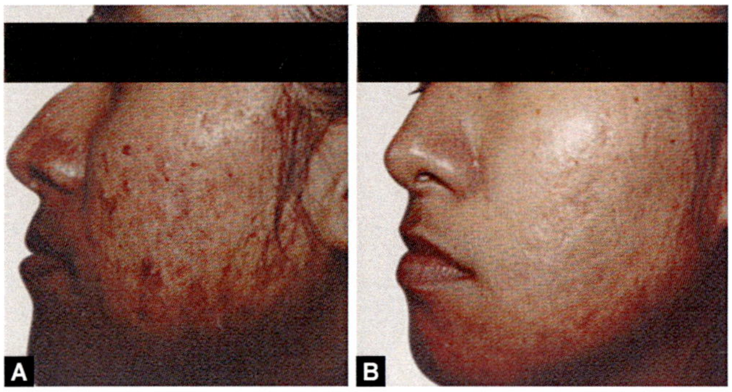

Figs 2.33A and B: Black acetic acid peel (A) Before and (B) after—28 years/female—6 sessions

- Apply black peel in even strokes. Single strokes
- Do not apply on upper and lower eyelid
- Application to be completed in approx 45 seconds
- 2nd coat can be applied only on acne spots if required
- Leave it for 3 minutes
- Neutralize peel
- Hydrating mask to be applied for 20 minutes
- Apply sunscreen after removing the mask
- It improves dyskeratosis and better tolerated than Jessner's peel, the advantage is this peel has quicker results in a week's time
- There might be slight irritation and redness for a week.

Post-peel Care

- Erythema may appear which will subside in 1-2 days
- Peeling starts on 3rd day which settles in a week
- Wash face with water after 12 hours
- Soap can be applied after 24 hours
- Apply sunscreen.

Treatment Protocol

- *Day 1:* Black peel is done
- *Day 8:* Acne spot treatment for a week
- *Day 16-21:* Break
- *Day 22:* 2nd Black peel.

3

CHAPTER

Micromesotherapy

INTRODUCTION (FIGS 3.1 AND 3.2)

It is a minimally invasive microinjection technique used to treat variety of cosmetic and medical conditions. Vitamins and antioxidants are perfused through microchannels (300,000 microchannels in 6 minutes) created on the skin by a special equipment known as Dermaroller/Mesopen. It stimulates the skin cells to produce and promote collagen and elastin deposition in the dermis, just below the surface of the skin.

The microneedles puncture the layer of the epidermis, which is the main obstruction to penetration of the active ingredients.

There are various delivery systems in microneedling, but microneedling via Mesopen system creates literally thousands of channels through the epidermis, appears to be the most-effective. Mesopen channelling method is safe, cost effective and simple. Needle depth is preset and cannot penetrate deeper than the length of the needles avoiding any possibilities of injury.

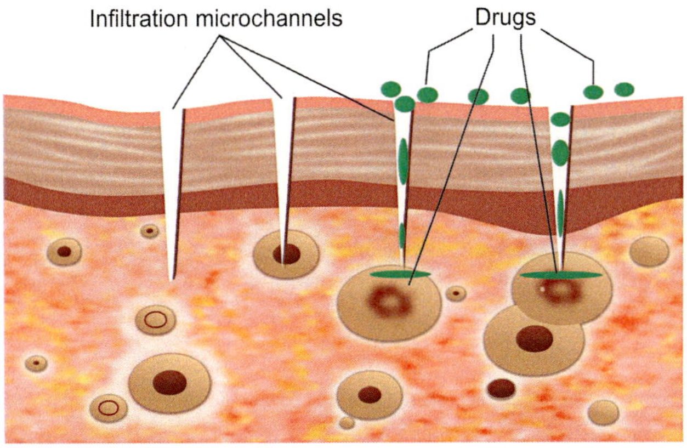

Fig. 3.1: Infiltration of vitamins and antioxidants via microchannels

INDICATIONS

- Scars due to acne, burns or trauma
- Resistant pigmentation
- Fine lines
- Open pores
- Stretch marks
- Hair follicle stimulation.

CONTRAINDICATIONS

- Active infection
- Chronic skin disorders
- Blood clotting disorders
- Uncontrolled diabetes
- Skin malignancies
- Active acne
- Solar keratosis
- Raised moles or warts
- Eczema
- Rosacea
- Psoriasis.

ADVANTAGES

- Treatment does not damage the skin
- Skin becomes thicker with greater than a 400% increase in collagen deposition and significantly more elastin
- Any part of the body can be treated
- May be safely done in people with darker pigmented skin, without fear of hyperpigmentation
- The skin does not become photosensitive
- The technique is easy to master using Dermaroller/Mesopen tool that has been specially designed for the procedure.

PROCEDURE

- Procedure must be explained to the client and informed consent taken in advance
- Take pictures before and after treatment
- Clean the skin with 70% isopropyl alcohol
- Apply topical anesthetic cream to the concerned area and leave it for about 45 minutes to 1 hour
- Choose a Dermaroller/Mesopen that fits the purpose of the treatment. Stretch the skin with one hand. With the other hand, start rolling the roller in one direction from left to right, top to bottom and diagonally distributing uniform force or create microchannels with a Mesopen. You must avoid imposing excessive stimulation on the eye area and cheek bones. Do not impose excessive pressure on the roller

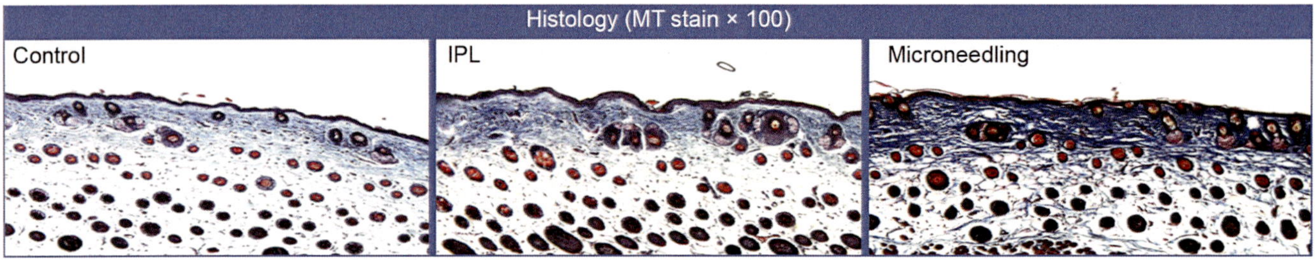

Fig. 3.2: Histology of microneedling

- Apply the drug or products containing the ingredients that will serve the treatment purposes evenly on the concerned area. The multiple holes created by needling will deliver the ingredients deep into the skin. Leave the drug or product for about 10 minutes for more effective infiltration
- Clean the area with the normal saline. Give cold saline compresses
- Apply antibiotic cream on treated area
- Apply sunscreen.

RESULTS OF SKIN NEEDLING (FIGS 3.3 TO 3.8)

Skin needling will increase the effectiveness of skin care products allowing improved penetration of vitamins and other active ingredients into the active layer of skin.

INDICATIONS OF USING DIFFERENT NEEDLE LENGTHS (FIG. 3.9)

- 0.5 mm needle length
  - Hair follicle stimulation
  - Mesoglow
- 1.0 mm
  - Facial rejuvenation
  - Pigment reduction
  - Fine lines and wrinkles
  - Photoaging

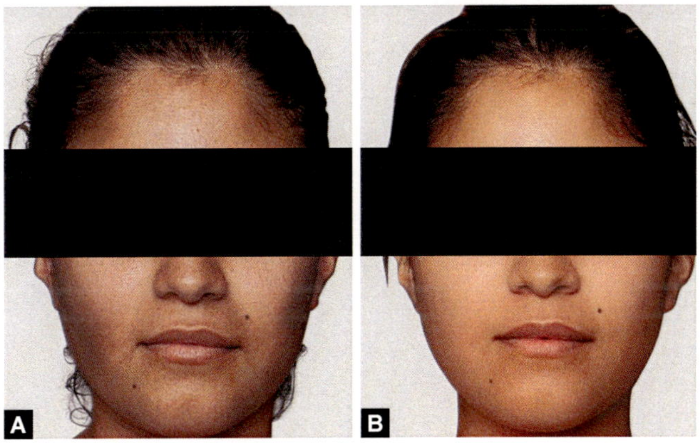

Figs 3.3A and B: Results of skin needling (A) Before and (B) after—29 years/female—5 sessions

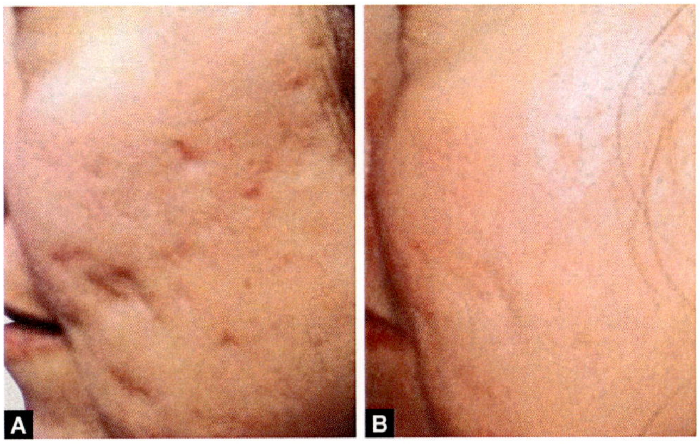

Figs 3.4A and B: Results of skin needling (A) Before and (B) after—55 years/female—5 sessions

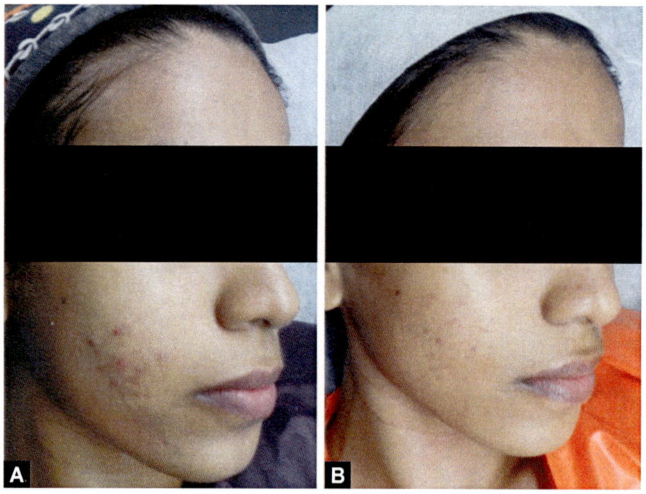

Figs 3.5A and B: Results of skin needling (A) Before and (B) after—27 years/female—5 sessions

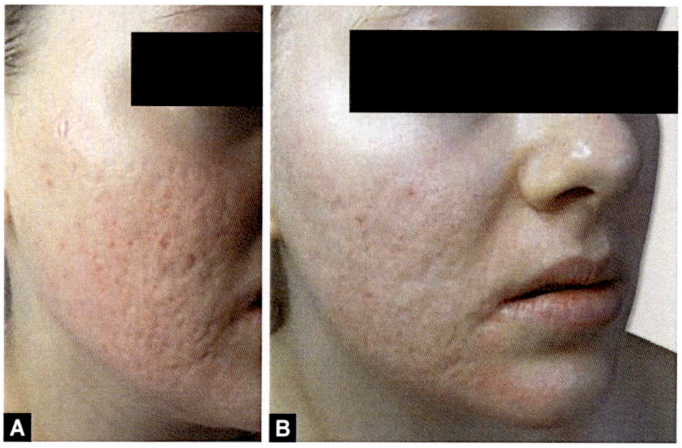

Figs 3.6A and B: Results of skin needling (A) Before and (B) after—33 years/female—5 sessions

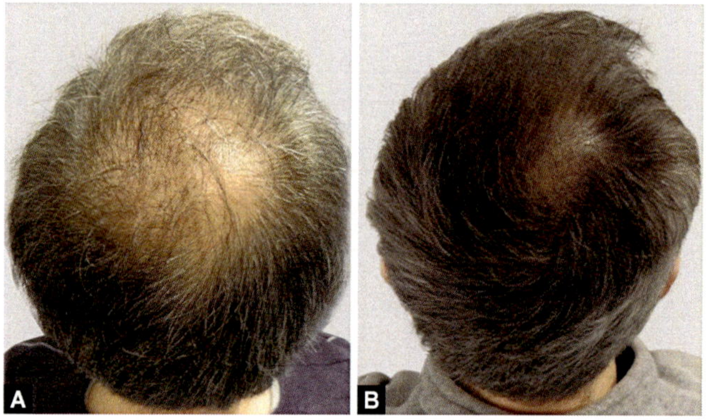

Figs 3.7A and B: Results of skin needling (A) Before and (B) after—34 years/male—12 sessions

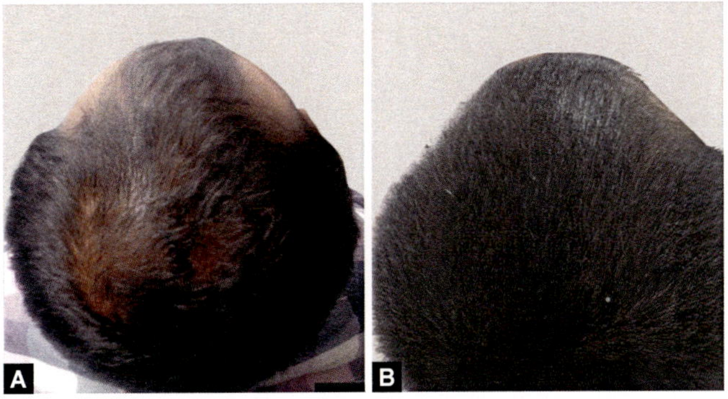

Figs 3.8A and B: Results of skin needling (A) Before and (B) after—28 years/male—10 sessions

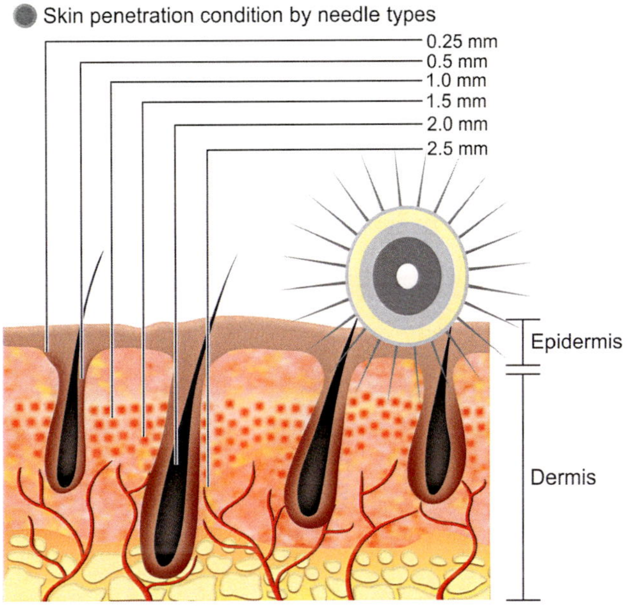

Fig. 3.9: Depth of needle in microneedling

- 1.5 mm/2.0 mm
  - Scar reduction
  - Stretch marks.

PRODUCTS USED IN MICROMESOTHERAPY

- *Scars:* Hyaluronic acid (1%), vitamin C
- *Pigmentation:* Glutathione, arbutin, vitamin C, Sulforawhite
- *Wrinkles:* Ameliox, hyaluronic acid, stem cells
- *Stretch marks:* DMAE (4%), Venofresh, *Ginkgo biloba*, silicon (5%), vitamin C
- *Skin rejuvenation:* CoQ10, stem cells, vitamins
- *Hair:* Pantothenic acid, biotin, *Ginkgo biloba*, Minoxidil, finasteride, dutasteride, anti-hair loss solution containing aminoacids, peptides, vitamins and minerals, stem cells.

Hyaluronic Acid

Hyaluronic acid promotes keratinocyte proliferation and migration and increases the penetration of retinoic acid, effecting skin hydration. It helps in collagen synthesis and normal skin function. Present in the extracellular matrix of basal keratinocytes, hyaluronic acid is critical to the structural integrity of the dermal collagen matrix. These benefits make hyaluronic acid a very effective topical humectant. It allows a fluid circulation of nutrients in the skin. It has moisturizing effect and maintains skin tone with anti-aging and lifting effect. It hydrates the skin by holding in water & contributes to dermal renewal.

Vitamin C

It is an effective skin antioxidant. It inhibits melanin production. It stabilizes oily, acne-prone skin. It gives a refreshed appearance and a radiant glow. It improves skin tone, boosts collagen and elastin production, smoothens and minimizes fine lines, scars, wrinkles. Reduces puffiness and helps aging. Vitamin C is used mainly to treat & prevent photoageing, uneven complexion along with treating the wrinkles.

Ameliox

Ameliox has two components:

1. Carnosine is a di-peptide which prevents cross-linking and stiffening of collagen by glycation. It relaxes the connective tissue, smoothens expression lines and rejuvenates. Carnosine is an endogenous anti-aging factor.
2. Silymarin prevents premature skin aging. It protects the skin against oxidative stress. It is an oil soluble antioxidant.

Co-enzyme Q10

It is found in every cell in the body and is important in the production of energy within each and every cell in the human body. It is essential for the health of cells, tissues and organs.

Co-enzyme Q10 has powerful antioxidant effects and destroys free radicals in the body. It helps the body's energy production in the form of ATP (adenosine triphosphate). It works in a synergistic way with vitamin E. It rejuvenates skin by enhancing cell efficiency.

Stem Cells

It shows a remarkable anti-hyaluronidase and anti-collagenase action that reduces deterioration of epidermal structural macromolecules, and encourages the skin's redensification and revitalization.

Minoxidil

It is an effective vasodilator. It is a K^+ channel opener thereby stimulating mitosis and enhancing the growth of suboptimal follicles. It is a 1–3% solution in a base of 10% propylene glycol, 20% distilled water and 70% alcohol. It converts vellus hairs to terminal ones in 30% cases.

Finasteride

It is a inhibitor of 5-alpha reductase (type II isoenzyme). It prevents conversion of testosterone to dihydrotestosterone (DHT). Peak plasma concentrations are achieved within first 2 hours of oral administration. Finasteride 1 mg/day causes reduction of serum DHT by 65%. Micromesotherapy with finasteride helps to minimize the side effects of long-term oral treatment and also reduces apprehension of clients.

Silicon

Silicon dissolves fibrotic bands seen in cellulite. It also stimulates collagen synthesis.

Sulforawhite

It deactivates reactive oxidants generated by ultraviolet (UV) rays in keratinocytes by stimulating the cellular antioxidant defense system.

Besides, it inhibits the binding of alpha-melanocyte stimulating hormone (α-MSH) on melanocytes. α-MSH is a hormone produced by pituitary gland which binds to receptors on melanocytes which stimulates cascade of events to induce skin pigmentation.

Arbutin

Arbutin is the active substance originated from a natural plant which can whiten and lighten skin. It can infiltrate into the skin quickly without affecting cell multiplication and effectively prevent activity of tyrosinase in the skin and the formation of melanin. By inhibiting tyrosinase, decomposition and drainage of melanin are accelerated and pigments can be reduced without any side effects.

Dimethylaminoethanol

Dimethylaminoethanol (DMAE) is a precursor of acetylcholine which acts as a stabilizer and an antioxidant on the cellular membrane, protecting it against organic stress. Acetylcholine, a neurotransmitter involved with muscle tone, improves the firmness and counteracts the flaccidity of skin. It increases skin elasticity and hydration with lifting effect.

Biotin

Biotin is known as vitamin B8 and vitamin H and plays an important role on the metabolism of carbohydrates, proteins and fats. It catalyzes the fixation of carbon dioxide in the synthesis of fatty acids. The root of the hair follicle has an active metabolism which is very sensitive to nutritional deficit of vitamins which can cause fragility and consequently hair loss. Biotin gives a revitalizing effect. It helps in hair regeneration.

Ginkgo Biloba

The leaf extract of *Ginkgo biloba*, increases collagen synthesis on the blood vessels walls. It protects collagen and hyaluronic acid. Useful on treatment for lipodystrophy associated with micro-circulation disorders.

Venofresh

It is a non-tensioactive substance that acts over the cellular membrane by decreasing the permeability of the sodium ions and when used at high concentrations also of potassium ions.

Glutathione

Glutathione has reducing group sulfhydryl (SH) which can form a complex with copper and inhibits tyrosinase activity. It also quenches free radicals and acts as a powerful antioxidant. It mediates the switch mechanism from eumelanogenesis to pheomelanogenesis.

4

CHAPTER

Mesotherapy

INTRODUCTION

Mesotherapy is a non-surgical cosmetic medical treatment. It is a painless procedure of injecting vitamins, minerals, medications, amino acids, stem cells and plant extracts placed in the dermis or subcutaneous tissue. It is a method of drug delivery.

MECHANISM OF ACTION

Mechanism of action of mesotherapy is that the solutions that are injected intracutaneously remain in the area longer than they would if delivered via deeper injection because they are cleared more slowly by the general circulation. In addition, it is felt that these superficially injected solutions continue to penetrate into the deeper tissues. The more superficial the injections, the longer the solution remains in the area.

Mesotherapy can be used as a supplement or an alternative to many antiaging regimens, including botox, laser resurfacing, peels, antioxidants, topical creams and face lifts.

Mesotherapy is a medical technique

1. It requires good medical knowledge and practice.
2. Diagnosis is essential, using tests.
3. The result of the treatment is not linked to the amount of drug given but to the choice of drug.
4. This requires precise pharmacological criteria.

Mesotherapy requires

1. Proper technique.
2. Suitable drug combinations.
3. A sensible indication.
4. A correct clinical assessment.

BENEFITS

- Treat solar damaged skin
- Reduce fine lines and wrinkles

- Restore youthful, radiant and healthy skin
- Improve dark circles
- Improve marks and scars
- Regrow hair
- Lighten hyperpigmented areas
- Improve stretch marks
- Dissolve fat from the cheeks, love handles and double chin
- Improve cellulite.

METHODS (FIGS 4.1 AND 4.2)

- Intraepidermal
- Papular
- Nappage
- Point by point.

Intraepidermal

The most superficial (1 mm deep) of all the techniques in which the basal layer of skin is not penetrated. Needle size of 27 to 31 gauges is used with the bevel oriented away from the skin and dragged along with light, positive pressure applied to the plunger. It is done in a grid pattern at 1-cm intervals over the entire affected area. Multiple injections of small doses of medications, in precise locations, in a single sitting are required. The benefits of mesogun include faster injections, precise dose delivery, consistent depth of penetration and more comfort for the physician and patient.

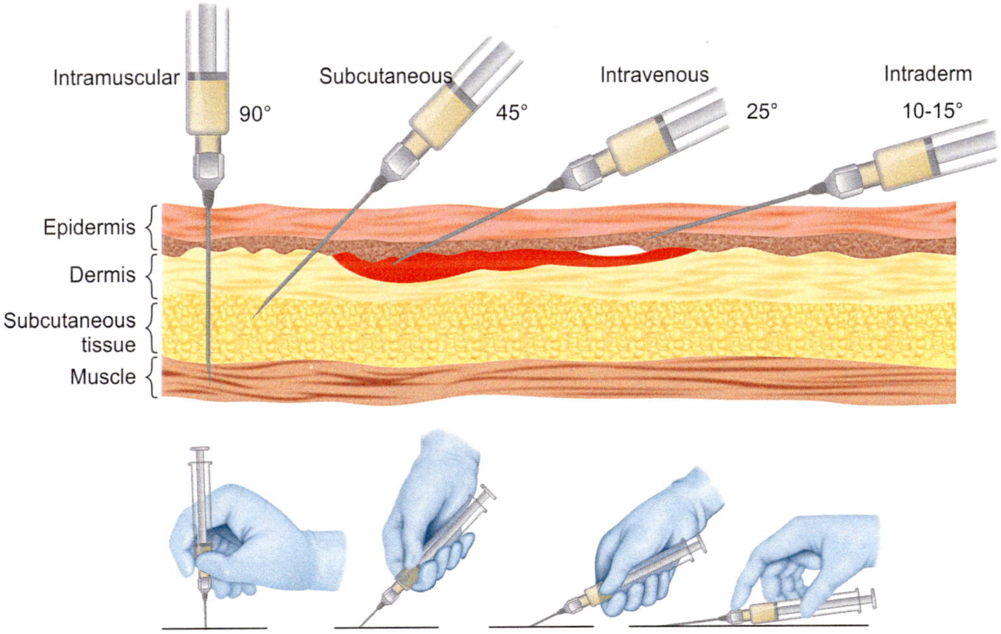

Fig. 4.1: Angle for inserting injection

- **Papule:**
  1–2 mm, with bevel upwards
- **Nappage:**
  2–4 mm, angle of 30°–60°
- **Point-by-boint**
  Deep injections, 4–12 mm

Fig. 4.2: Injection technique

Papule

A superficial intradermal technique, which consists of injecting the product at the junction between epidermis and dermis, not penetrating the basal lamina. Tip of the needle is inserted into the most superficial layer at a depth of 1–2 mm, with bevel facing upwards. A pale, clearly delineated papule appears at the time of injection and disappears within 30 minutes. Suitable for wrinkles and immunostimulation.

Nappage (French for "Covering")

Involves more superficial (2 mm deep) injections with a 4-mm needle, covering a large area. Injections are given at a 45 degree angle from the skin while applying light, constant positive pressure on the plunger, the practitioner rapidly flicks the wrist (mimics shaking a salt shaker or the action of a sewing machine). At each site, a drop of solution is introduced. Relatively, this is a more discomforting procedure to the patient.

Point by Point

First described by Dr. Pistor, involves injection of 0.02 mL to 0.05 mL of drug solution. It is deep intradermal or hypodermic injection technique, consisting of separate injections at depths from 4–12 mm or even 15 mm depending on the area. Injection should be given 1–2 cm apart (Fig. 4.3).

USES

The medical benefits include improved blood flow to the area, dissolving excess fat deposits, removing fibrotic, hardened connective tissue and improving lymphatic drainage.

STEPS

- Precleansing
- Marking
- Injecting
- Postcleansing.

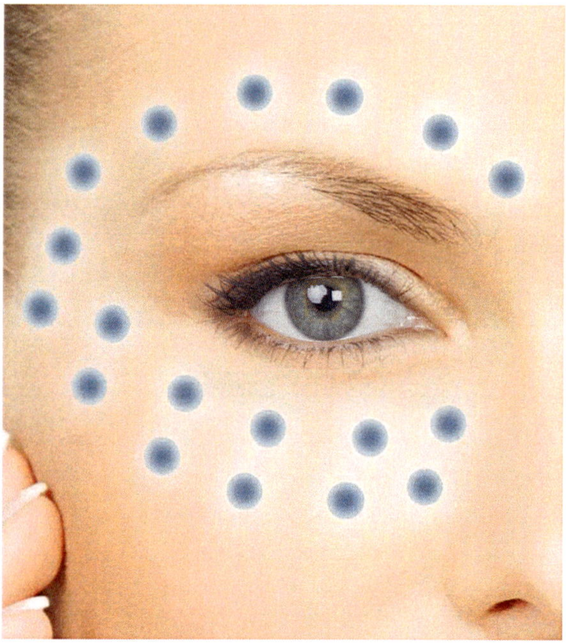

Fig. 4.3: Point-by-point injection

NUMBER OF SESSIONS REQUIRED

- Generally the average patient requires 4–5 treatments
- *Facial Areas:* After three weeks
- *Other Parts:* Alternate week.

DIFFERENT TYPES OF MESO TREATMENTS

Mesoglow (Fig. 4.4)

Mesoglow is a series of microinjections injected onto the skin. It consists of injecting products designed to revitalize the skin and give it a refreshing natural glow. It is a procedure to reduce the signs of ageing. It provides hydration and nutrients by placing droplets into the skin by nappage technique, thus starting the rejuvenation process. Mesoglow rejuvenates and revives dull, tired skin, to give youthful and glowing appearance.

The benefits of skin rejuvenation can be long lasting. If one practices overall good health, the effects can last one year otherwise treatments are needed in six months.

Eye Rejuvenation (Fig. 4.5)

It is consists of microinjections into the skin, which significantly contributes to cell proliferation, migration and tissue repair. Reduces pigmentation and prevents fine lines and wrinkles by generating new skin cells and hydrates dry skin. To get good results progressive sessions of 5–6 treatments are done 1 week apart.

VAMPIRE FACELIFT®

Vampire facelift, also known as rich plasma therapy, aims to rejuvenate the skin by injecting blood in the skin. It is also called platlet rich plasma (PRP) therapy. The person's own blood is taken and platelet-rich plasma is separated. Vitamins and amino acids are then mixed and serum is injected into the face to bring about improvements in premature aged skin and bring about younger look. It can be done by nappage technique or point by point technique.

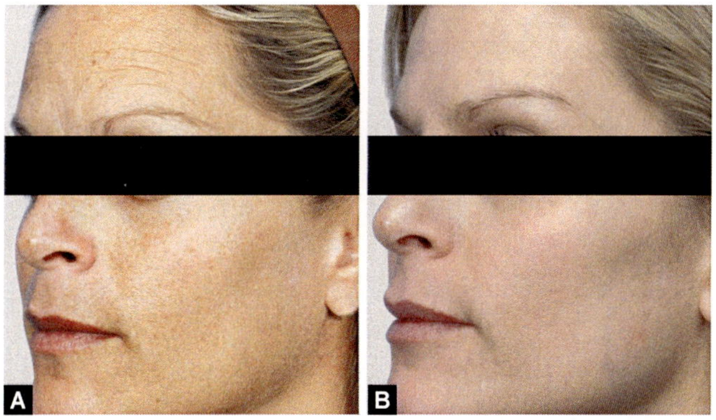

Figs 4.4A and B: Mesoglow (A) Before and (B) after—Mesoglow—32 years/female—5 sessions

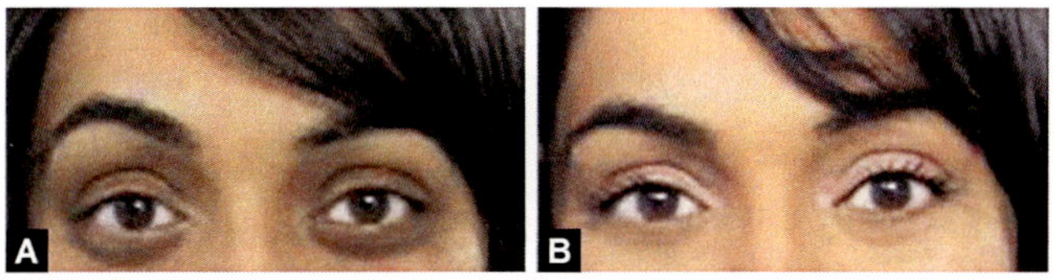

Figs 4.5A and B: Eye rejuvenation (A) Before and (B) after—Mesoglow and puffy eyes—32 years/female—5 sessions

Cellulite Treatment

A cellulite mesotherapy treatment requires at least 3 months time. In treating cellulite, for better clinical results, it is important to use a combination of different techniques, including mesotherapy. To be effective, these techniques have to work first on the extra cellular matrix, the microcirculation (arteriolar, capillary, venous) and the lymphatic system, and finally, on the fat tissue. It is done by point by point technique.

SIDE EFFECTS

A common side effect of mesotherapy is bruising, which generally resolves over one week. Patients may experience temporary soreness. This will subside within 24–48 hours. Preparation generally takes 30 minutes and requires no recovery time. Maintenance required once a month.

5

CHAPTER

Platelet-rich Plasma

INTRODUCTION

Platelet-rich plasma (PRP) has been used in many medical fraternities like orthopedic medicine, dentistry, and reconstructive surgery, and now it is becoming popular in dermatology for skin, wound healing, melasma and pigmentation, hair growth and scalp rejuvenation. It is a nonsurgical cosmetic medicine treatment, which includes multiple microinjections of PRP product into the mesodermal layer of the skin. Scientific studies have documented that PRP grows new collagen when injected into the skin, and it works very well as an alternative tool for antiaging. Various methods have been tested for clinical use of PRP in skin rejuvenation, such as the traditional method, buffy-coat method, the plasma separator method, etc. Some of these methods are discussed in detail below. Ready kits are available for the buffy-coat method and plasmolifting in the market today.

COMPONENTS

The efficacy of certain growth factors and the concentrations of the same found within PRP are the theoretical basis for its use in tissue repair. The PRP is activated by addition of thrombin and calcium chloride, which induces the release of the below mentioned factors from alpha granules. The growth factors and other cytokines present in PRP include the following:

- Platelet-derived growth factor
- Transforming growth factor beta
- Fibroblast growth factor
- Insulin-like growth factor 1
- Insulin-like growth factor 2
- Vascular endothelial growth factor
- Epidermal growth factor
- Interleukin 8
- Keratinocyte growth factor
- Connective tissue growth factor.

PREPARATION OF ACTIVATED PRP

In the last couple of years, there have been two PRP preparation methods approved by the US. Food and Drug Administration. Both processes involve the collection of the patient's whole blood (that is anticoagulated with citrate dextrose) before undergoing two stages of centrifugation designed to separate the PRP from platelet-poor plasma and red blood cells. In humans, the typical baseline blood platelet count is approximately 2,00,000 per microliter, therapeutic PRP concentrates the platelets by roughly five-fold. The growth in platelet count differs depending on the technology and procedure variations.

Sample Collection For PRP

- Make the patient lie on the bed, wear gloves, prepare a 20 mL syringe with 20G/18G needle and flush it with sodium citrate/ACDA
- Prepare 1 sterile plastic container, flush it with saline and add about 2 mL of sodium citrate/ACDA each.
- Discover a prominent vein preferably from cubical area of elbow; clean the area with alcohol swab in circular fashion from inside to outside
- Withdraw about 18 mL of blood, while withdrawing do not move your hand (it might cause counter of vein)
- Place the withdrawn blood in a sterile container
- Meanwhile ask the person who is assisting you to press the withdrawal site with a cotton piece for about 1 minute or until the bleeding stops, apply a fresh band aid at that site.

PRP Procedure 1 (Figs 5.1 and 5.2)

Explain procedure to the client.

- Take informed consent form duly signed by the patient
- Clean the face with cleanser according to skin type
- Pictures to be taken for before and after record
- Follow the sample collection steps mentioned above
- After putting blood in vial containing ACDA/sodium citrate, start centrifugation procedure for 5–10 minutes at frequency 1000–1500 RPM for 10 minutes
- Separate yellow plasma (supernatant) and take in another vial
- The new vial containing PRP to be kept in centrifugation machine for heavy spin at frequency of 3000 rpm for 10–12 minutes

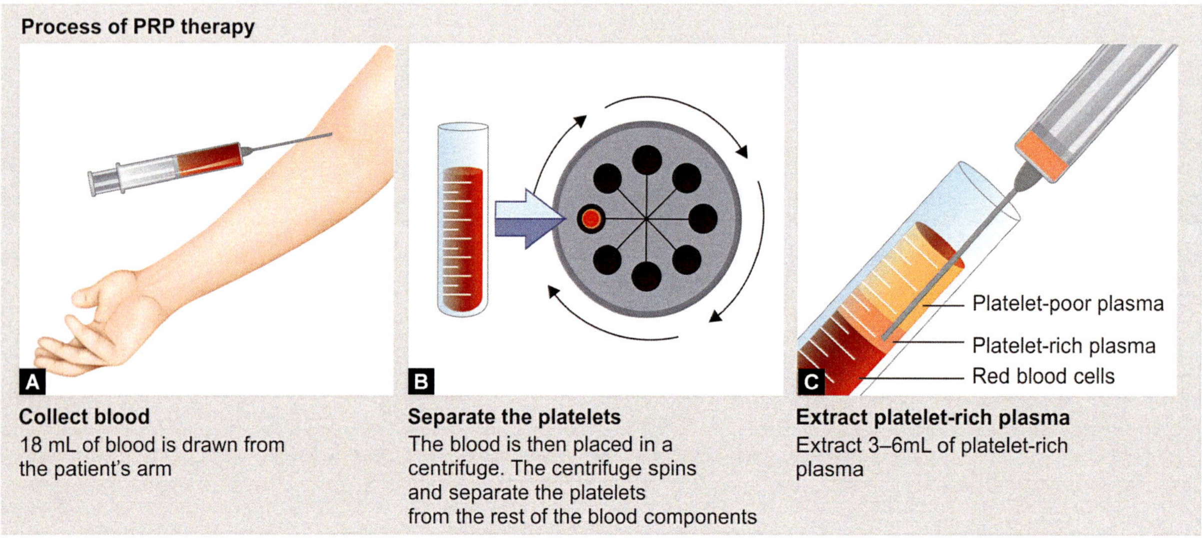

Figs 5.1 A to C: PRP method

- Inject as soon as possible with help of insulin syringes
- Direct intradermal injections of 0.01–0.02 mL/cm^2 are given in a retrograde fashion from deep to superficial, at every centimeter, throughout the treated site
- As an adjuvant to laser or microneedling it is usually done once in every 3–6 months for 1 year and then yearly as maintenance (Figs 5.3 to 5.5).

The second type of procedure which is widely practiced is plasmolifting using a plasma separator kit. In this procedure 8 mL of blood with 2 mL of anticoagulant (already present in tube) is withdrawn in plasma separator kit and centrifuged only once. After centrifuging we get 3–4 mL of plasma which is rich in growth factors. This entire plasma is injected with insulin syringes.

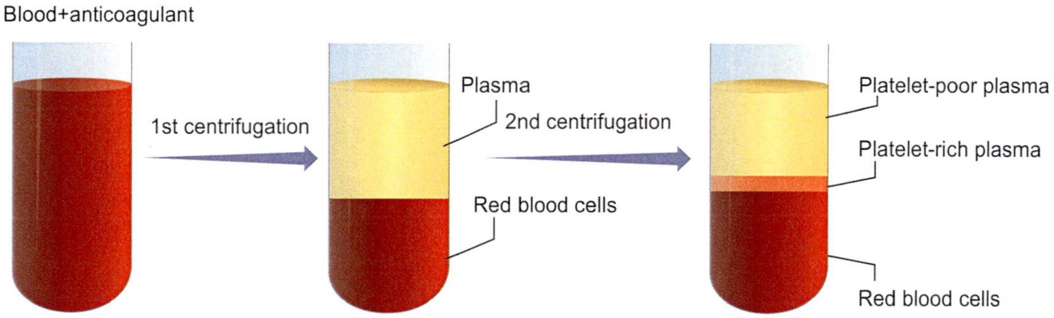

Fig. 5.2: Buffy-coat method

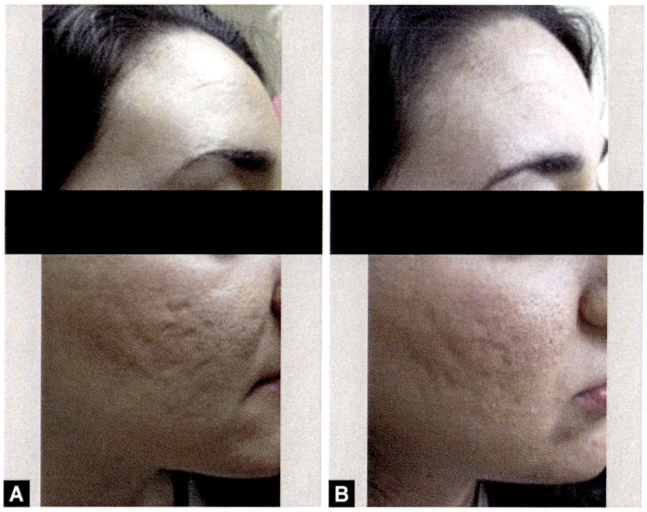

Figs 5.3A and B: (A) Before and (B) after—34 years/female—3 sessions

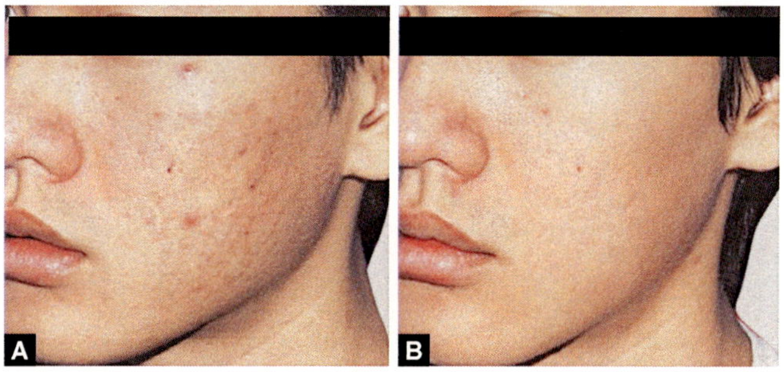

Figs 5.4A and B: (A) Before and (B) after—25 years/male—3 sessions

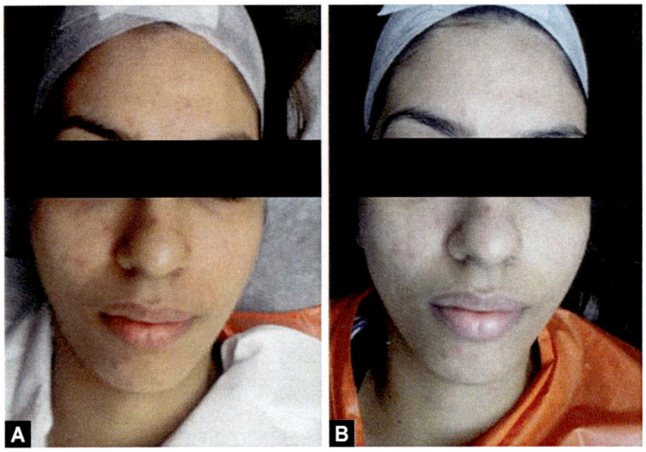

Figs 5.5A and B: (A) Before and (B) after—25 years / female—3 sessions

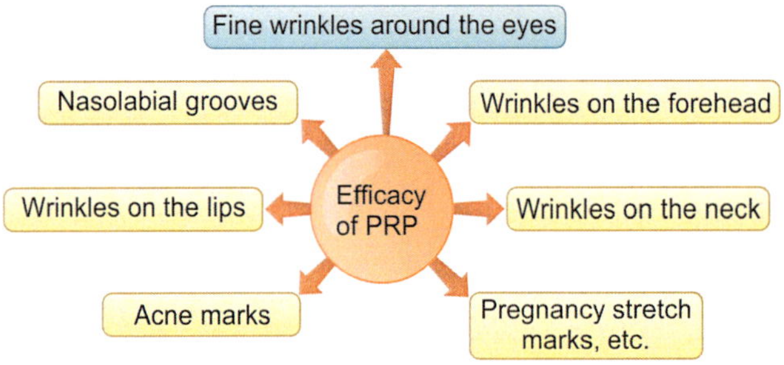

Fig 5.6: Indications

INDICATIONS (FIG 5.6)

- Facial rejuvenation
- Acne scars and contour defects
- Anti-aging
  - Wrinkles—Face, lips, neck and hands
  - Loose and saggy skin
- Nasolabial grooves
- Dark circles and eye bags
- Stretch marks
- Hair regeneration and restoration
- Lipodermatosclerosis
- Lichen sclerosus.

MODE OF ACTION IN SKIN REJUVENATION

- Increased proliferation of human dermal fibroblast
- Increased production of collagen type I peptide and expression of collagen type I, alpha-I leading to synthesis of new collagen
- Increases expression of G1 cell cycle regulators which accelerates wound healing.

CONTRAINDICATIONS

- H/O of heavy smoking, drug and alcohol use
- Platelet dysfunction syndrome

- Thrombocytopenias
- Hypofibrinogenemia
- Hemodynamic instability
- Sepsis, acute and chronic infections
- Chronic liver diseases
- Anti-coagulation therapy
- Chronic skin diseases or cancer
- Metabolic and systemic disorders.

CONCLUSION

Monthly intradermal injections of PRP in 3 sessions shows satisfactory result in face and neck rejuvenation and hair restoration. PRP can be combined with other non-ablative procedures like erbium glass laser, other fractional lasers and micromesotherapy. The goal of PRP skin rejuvenation therapy is to improve skin tone and texture, tighten skin, soften lines and pores. There is objective improvement in skin elasticity and increase in collagen density as well.

PRP injections given monthly for 3 months give good results for infraorbital rejuvenation as well without any obvious side effects. The injection of PRP is a safe, painless and less time consuming process with minimal downtime.

In summary, face and neck revitalization with PRP is a promising, easy-to-use technique, performed favorably in fine lines, wrinkles, scars. Good results were also observed to improve uneven skin tone, texture and elasticity. PRP is derived from our own blood cells, eliminating the possibility of negative side effects. The technique has been accepted and practiced by industry experts. Objective clinical results were good. Patient's satisfaction and feedback was good. The technique's exact mechanism of action has not yet been entirely clarified. Although the method needs further validations, initial results are encouraging and promising.

6

CHAPTER

Botulinum Toxin

INTRODUCTION

As we age, our faces begin to show the effects of gravity, sun exposure and years of facial muscle movement, such as smiling, chewing and squinting.

The underlying tissues that keep our skin looking youthful and plumped up begin to break down, often leaving behind laugh lines, smile lines, crow's feet or facial creases over the areas where this excessive muscle movement occurs.

Botulinum toxin is a natural protein, which relaxes the muscles causing wrinkles creating a smooth and youthful appearance. It is an extract from bacteria in a highly purified form. It is one of the most gratifying procedures in practice. It is a common cosmetic procedure amongst all cosmetic procedures effective for both men and women. It is affordable as compared to appearance-related investments like wrinkle creams, hair coloring and facials. It does not change the radical appearance like a face-lift would do. It remains in the sight of injection and its results last for about 3–6 months.

MECHANISM OF ACTION

Botulinum toxin contains a protein complex purified from the bacterium *Clostridium botulinum.* A component of this complex, Botulinum Toxin Type A is the important active ingredient. Type A is one of the seven distinct botulinum toxins produced by different strains of the bacterium. Botulinum toxin decreases muscle activity by blocking overactive nerve impulses that trigger excessive muscle contractions or glandular activity.

Phase I—Nerve-Muscle Communication is Blocked

Botulinum toxin blocks the transmission of overactive nerve impulses to the targeted muscle by selectively preventing the release of the neurotransmitter acetylcholine (ACh) at the neuromuscular junction, temporarily preventing muscle contraction. This is primarily a local effect. Botulinum toxin is also injected into the skin to treat the symptoms of severe underarm sweating (severe primary axillary hyperhidrosis) when medicines used on the skin (topical) do not work well enough in people 18 years and older. Botulinum toxin is a prescribed medicine that is injected into muscles and used to improve the look of moderate to severe lines between the eyebrows in people 18–65 years of age for a short period of time (temporary).

Binding

The heavy chain portion of the active ingredient in botulinum toxin (onabotulinumtoxinA) neurotoxin binds to the cell membrane of the motor nerve via an unidentified high affinity "acceptor" molecule. This high affinity binding action allows for efficient uptake of botulinum toxin by the motor nerve and facilitates selective, targeted treatment at the injection site (Fig. 6.1).

Internalizing

After binding, the botulinum toxin protein molecule passes through the cell membrane of the motor nerve and into its cytoplasm via a process called endocytosis. It is here that the enzymatic component (light chain) of the botulinum toxin protein molecule is activated (Fig. 6.2).

Blocking

Inside the motor nerve, the light chain of the botulinum toxin (onabotulinumtoxinA) protein molecule cleaves apart a protein (called SNAP-25) that enables vesicles which store the neurotransmitter acetylcholine to attach to the cell membrane. Cleaving SNAP-25 prevents these vesicles from fusing with the membrane and prevents the release of acetylcholine into the neuromuscular junction (the space between the motor nerve and the muscle). Thus, nerve impulses that control muscle contractions are blocked decreasing muscle activity (Fig. 6.3).

Phase II—Nerve-Muscle Communication is Restored

The effect of botulinum toxin is generally temporary. Previous nerve impulse activity and associated muscle contractions resume over the course of a few to several months, depending on the individual patient and the indication for which they are being treated.

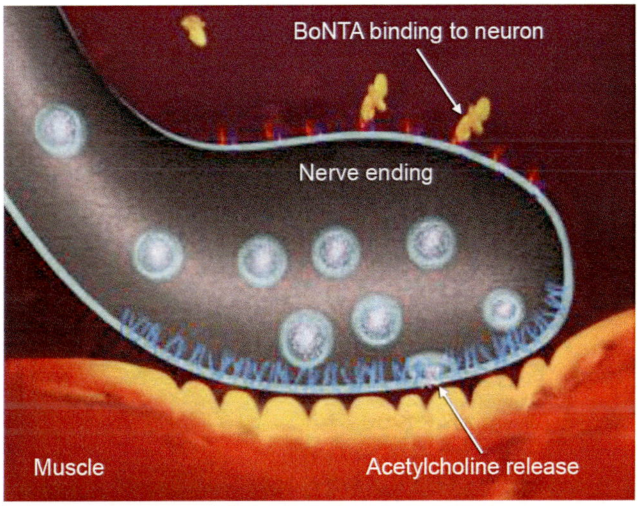

Fig. 6.1: Type A botulinum toxin action

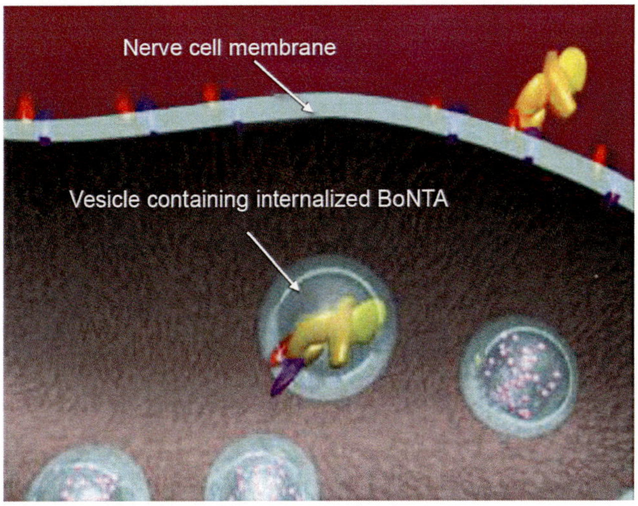

Fig. 6.2: Internalizing

Nerve Sprouting

New nerve endings sprout and connect to the muscle after the original nerve ending is blocked, renewing the ability of the nerve to cause muscle contractions (Fig. 6.4).

Original Nerve Connection Re-established

Eventually, the new nerve sprouts retract and the original nerve ending regains its function, suggesting that treatment with botulinum toxin (onabotulinumtoxinA) neurotoxin does not permanently alter the neuromuscular junction (Fig. 6.5).

RECONSTITUTION (TABLE 6.1)

- It is available in glass vials of 100 units and 50 units, which is a vacuum dried product. It must be stored at or below -5C. To reconstitute 100 units, 2.5 cc of preservative-free normal saline (0.9% sodium chloride) is injected into the vial and "gently" rotated. Do not shake the vial
- One must record the date and time of reconstitution
- Storage should be in the refrigerator and not the freezer because if ice crystals form the toxin is damaged and its potency decreases. Storage time is usually 4 weeks after reconstitution under ideal conditions.

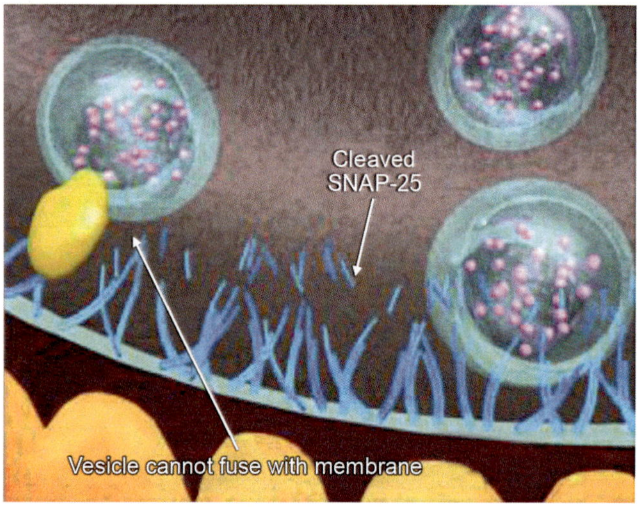

Fig. 6.3: Blocking

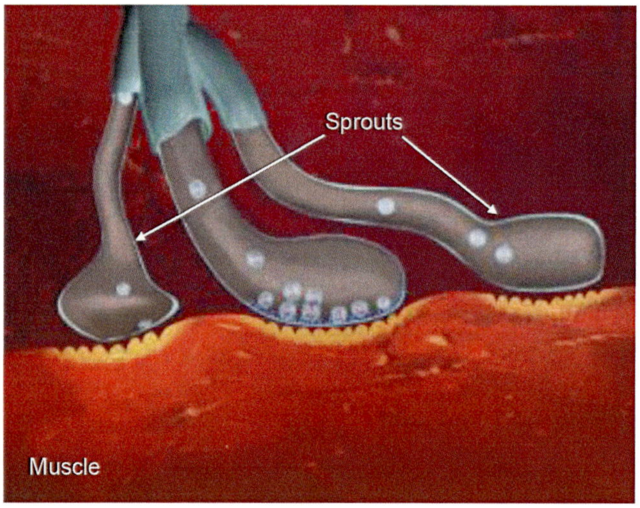

Fig. 6.4: Sprouting

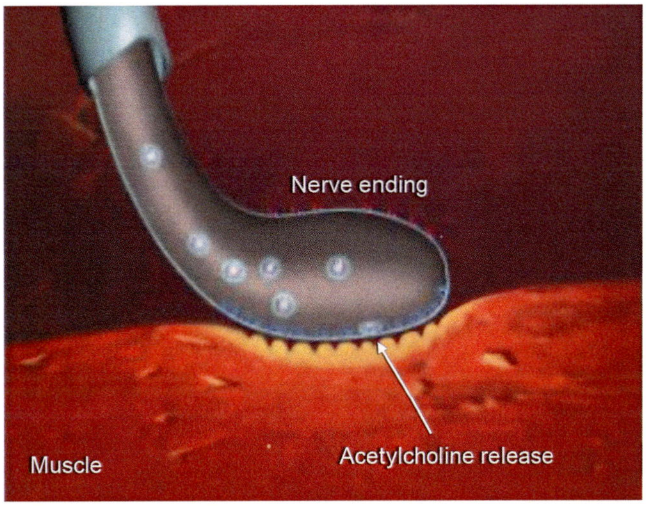

Fig. 6.5: Original nerve ending connection re-established

TABLE 6.1: Dilution instruction for botulinum toxin

Unit vial	*Diluents added (0.9% sodium chloride Injection)*	*Resulting dose (Units per 0.1 mL)*
50—unit vial	1.25 mL	4.00 units
100—unit vial	2.50 mL	4.00 units

Factors that may decrease potency are as follows:
- Alcohol on the skin or bottle cap
- Bubbles formed by foaming
- Agitation of bottle and syringe
- Storage time of diluted toxin.

ANATOMY OF FACIAL MUSCLES (TABLE 6.2 AND FIG. 6.6)

TABLE 6.2: List of muscles

Step No.	*Muscle involves*	*Function of the muscle*	*Function*
1.	Frontalis	Across forehead	Raises the eyebrows, draws scalp forward and wrinkles the forehead
2.	Procerus	Covers the top of the nose	Depresses the eyebrows and causes wrinkles across the bridge of the nose
3.	Corrugators	Beneath the frontalis and orbicularis oculi	Draws the eyebrows down and in. It produces vertical lines and causes frowning
4.	Orbicularis oculi	Completely surrounds the eye sockets	Closes the eyes
5.	Risorius and buccinator	Risorius—extends from masseter to the angle of the mouth Buccinator—between the upper and lower jaw	Risorius—draws down the corner of the mouth out and back as in grinning Buccinator—compresses cheeks and expels air between the lips as in blowing
6.	Masseter	From cheek bone to the outer side of the jaw	Coordinates in opening and closing of the mouth (chewing muscles)
7.	Orbicularis oris	Forms a flat band around upper and lower lip	Raises and draws back the upper lip and elevates the nostrils as in expressing distaste

Contd...

Contd...

Step No.	Muscle involves	Function of the muscle	Function
8.	Mentalis	Situated at the tip of the chin	Raises and pushes up the lower lip, causing wrinkling of the chin as in doubt or displeasure
9.	Platysma	Broad muscle that extends from the chest and shoulder muscle to the side of the chin	Depresses the lower jaw and lip as in the expression of sadness
10.	Sternocleidomastoid	Extends from the collar and chest bone to the temporal bone in the back of the ear	Rotates the head, also bends the head as in nodding

INDICATIONS (FIG. 6.7)

Basic

- Frown lines
- Horizontal forehead wrinkles
- Crow's feet
- Excessive sweating (hyperhidrosis).

Advanced

- Nasolabial folds and perioral lines
- Neck lines (Nefertiti lift, platysmal bands)
- Popply chin
- Mental crease
- Facial asymmetry.

Others

- Migraine (blepharospasm)
- Bunny lines
- Repeated nasal flare.

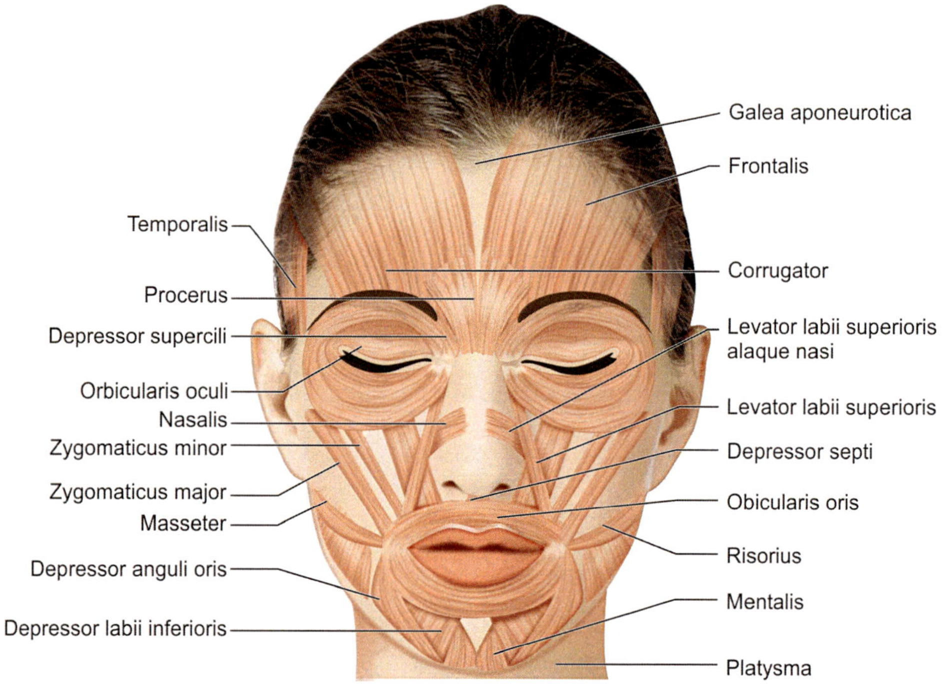

Fig. 6.6: Anatomy of facial muscles

CONTRADICTIONS

- Muscle disorders
- Epilepsy
- Pregnancy
- Breastfeeding
- Neuromuscular diseases.

METHODS

Before beginning the procedure confirm that the patient is not on any of the drugs like aspirin, warfarin, aminoglycosides. Give them a realistic idea via counseling. Take before and after photographs. Take written consent of the patient. Apply a topical anesthetic cream under occlusion (prilox, emla) 1 hour before the procedure.

Ask the patient to sit comfortable. Wipe the area to be injected with isopropyl alcohol and allow it to dry. Ask the patient to contract the muscles and mark the injection sites. The injection should be given 1 cm above the brow and 1 cm away from the orbital bony margin. For the forehead refer to the diagram above. Use a 30-gauge needle and insulin syringe. Calculate how much will be required for each area and inject 2–4 units per site as required. Male patients may require more units and more injection sites as the muscle mass is larger (Fig. 6.8).

OBSERVATIONS AND INSTRUCTIONS

Results begin to show in 2–3 days and the full effect is seen in a week.

- The effect lasts for 4–6 months. With successive treatments effect lasts for long
- It has been used for dynamic expression lines
- It is better to under correct than to overcorrect
- Patient should be called back after 2 weeks for a touch-up session if required
- It has a preventive effect on further deepening of the facial wrinkles
- It can be used on the lower half of the face but requires greater expertise.

SIDE EFFECTS

It is only seen if proper assessment and proper care while injecting is not done. Side effects are usually temporary and localized.

- Excessive arching of eyebrows
- Asymmetry
- Ptosis
- Bruising
- Tolerance
- Headache.

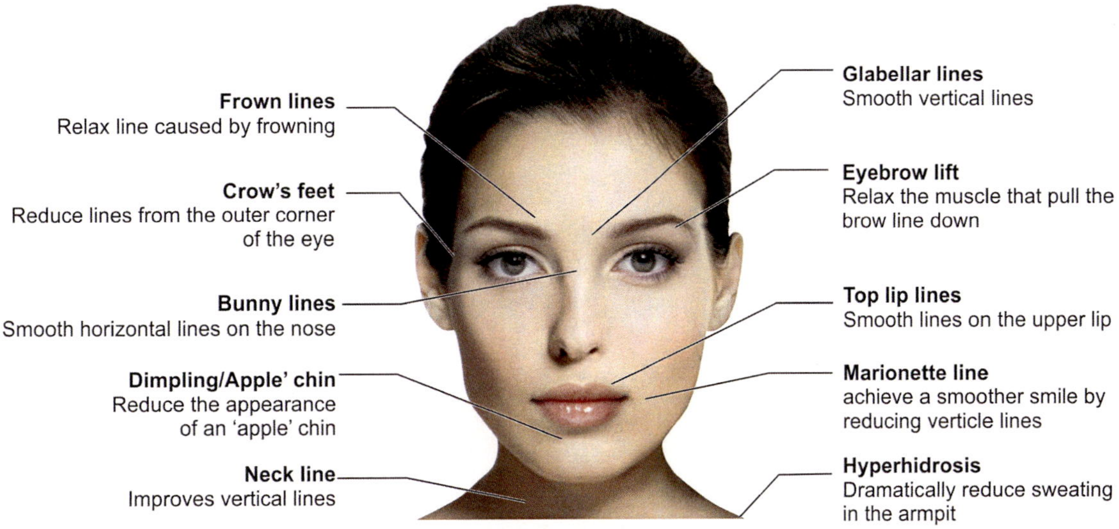

Fig. 6.7: Indications of botulinum toxin

COMBINATION TECHNIQUES

It could be combined with fillers, nonsurgical face-lift, glycolic peels, microdermabrasion, photo facials, etc. to enhance and rejuvenate overall appearance.

For example, if a patient has static frown lines first botulinum toxin is injected to smoothen the lines and then filler is injected 2 weeks later into the static line.

BASIC BOTULINUM TOXIN TECHNIQUES

1. *Horizontal lines:* The frontalis muscle elevates the brow and is associated with the development of horizontal forehead rhytides. 4-6 injection sites are recommended. Regardless of the number of injection sites it is important to remain 1-2 cm above orbital rim to reduce potential for brow ptosis. Maximum dose recommended for horizontal lines is 10-16 units. Reason for brow ptosis is overtreatment with botulinum toxin of the frontalis muscle. It results from overtreating the entire frontalis muscle within one finger breadth or 1-2 cm of the eyebrow. Avoid injecting 1cm above the brow to reduce brow ptosis. Do not treat the forehead (only glabellar and crow's feet) in patients over 60 who use frontalis to elevate the brow for better vision (Figs 6.9 and 6.10).

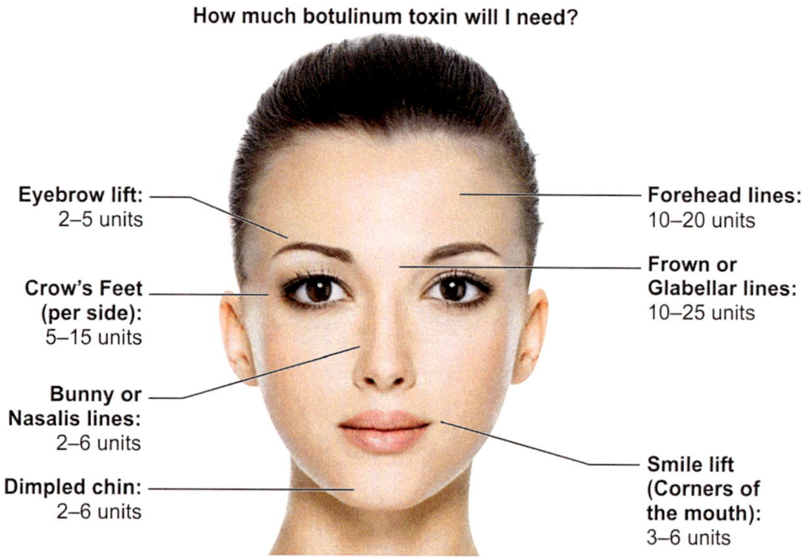

Fig. 6.8: Diagram indicative of units required per area

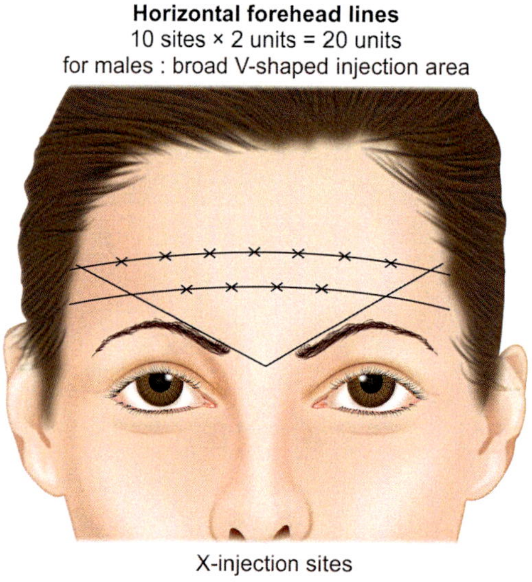

Fig. 6.9: Horizontal lines

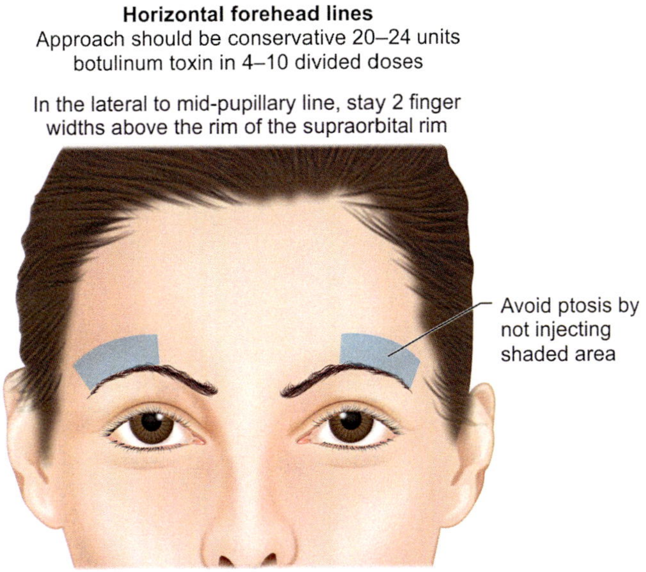

Fig. 6.10: Area to be avoided for ptosis

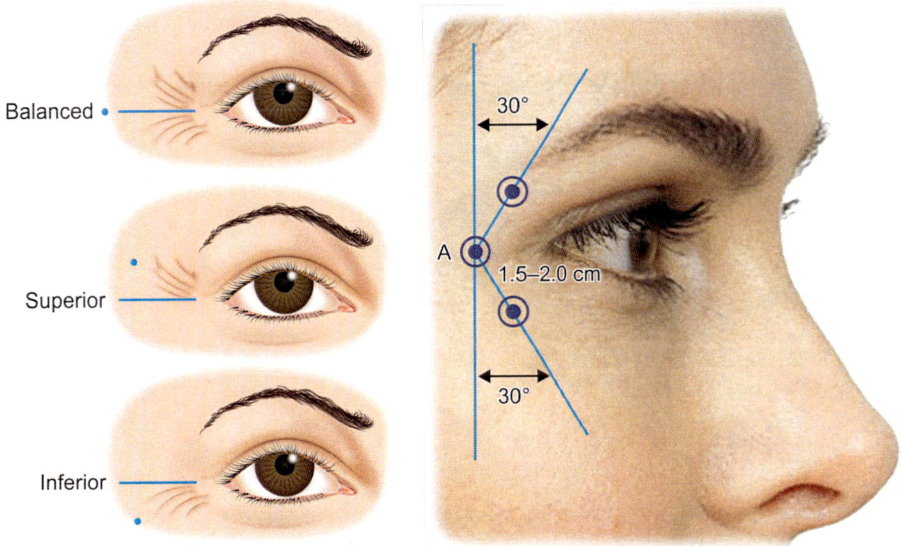

Figs 6.11A and B: Crow's feet (A) muscles and (B) injection points

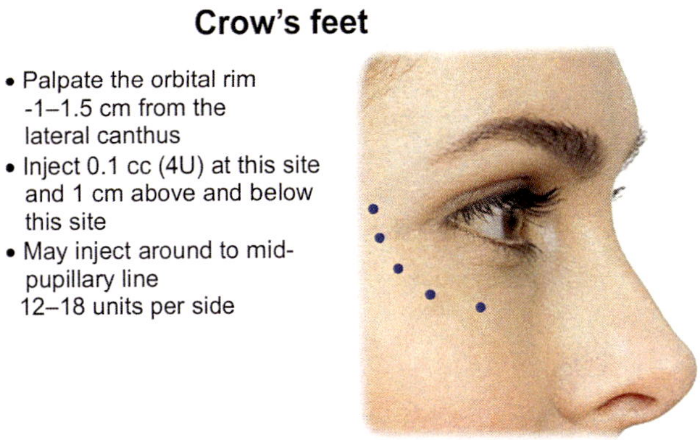

Fig. 6.12: Crow's feet

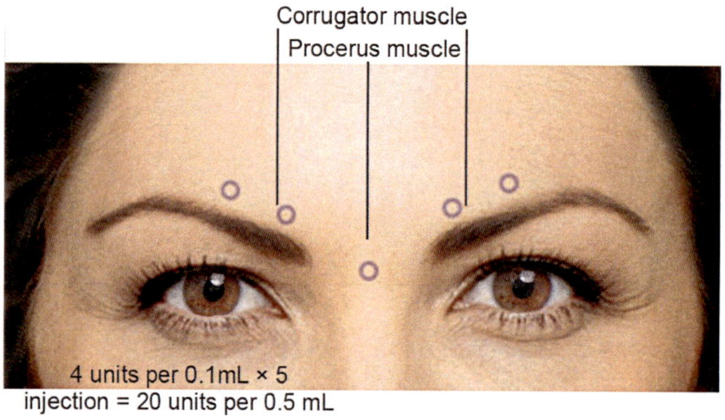

Fig. 6.13: Glabellar complex muscles

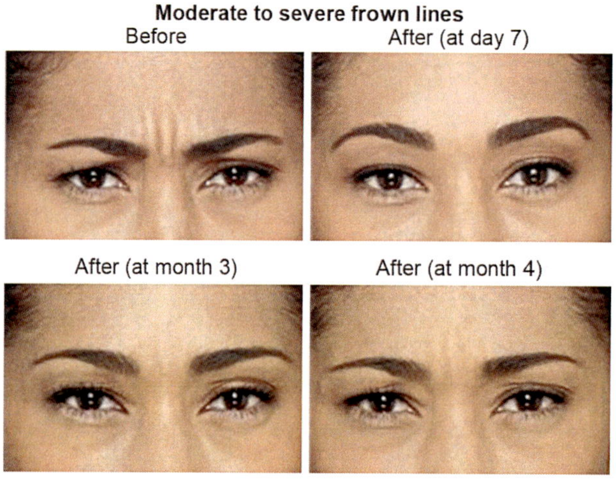

Fig. 6.14: Before and after – 34 years/female – Correction of glabellar complex

2. *Crow's feet:* Lateral orbital wrinkles called as crow's feet result from muscle activity along with photoageing. The treatment goal is to soften the wrinkles and provide relaxed look and not to cause immobility. The lateral fibers of orbicularis oculi are injected. On an average, 3-5 sites are injected on each side. The injection site is kept 1-1.5 cm lateral to the orbital rim. The second and third injection sites are approx 1-1.5 cm above and below the first injection site respectively. Regardless of distribution of crow's feet, the most anterior injection should be placed lateral to a line drawn vertically from the lateral canthus. The injections should be performed when the patient is not smiling as the toxin may affect the ipsilateral zygomaticus complex, causing ptosis of the upper lip. Maximum dose per side is 12-14 units. Should be done for patients who perform well to a preinjection snap test (lower eyelid briefly pulled off the globe by downward pressure on the lower eyelid skin, then quickly released, and the speed with which the eyelid snaps back to the globe assessed) (Figs 6.11 and 6.12).
3. *Glabellar complex:* The musculature of glabellar complex are corrugator supercilii, the procerus and depressor supercilii. Medial fibers of orbicularis oculi and frontalis can contribute as they interdigitate with the fibers of corrugator. 3-5 injection sites are recommended. Additional bilateral points above supraorbital rim at the mid-pupillary line may be considered. Injection sites depend on gender as male muscle mass is larger. Men tend to have a horizontal arch as against females who have gentle curved arch. Maximum dose for glabellar complex is 25 units (Figs 6.13 and 6.14).

7

CHAPTER

Advanced Botulinum Toxin Techniques

Mid- and lower-face botulinum toxin should be included in the therapeutic armamentarium of a doctor who is already experienced in the indications for upper face.

1. *Perioral lines/Smoker's lines:* Repeated purse string action of orbicularis oris leads to perioral lines. 1–2 units of botulinum toxin per lip quadrant is sufficient to give cosmetic benefit without creating paresis of orbicularis oris that might interfere with elocution and suction (Fig. 7.1).

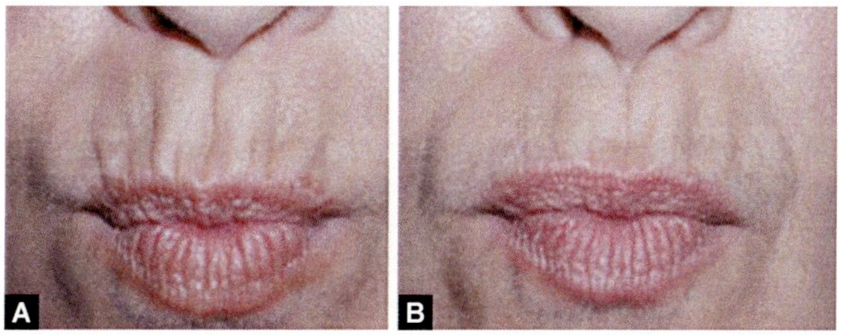

Figs 7.1A and B: (A) Before and (B) after—42 years/female—correction of perioral lines

2. *Nefertiti lift (horizontal lines):* These are the muscular subaponeurotic system attachments in the neck. Simplest approach is to dance along the lines injecting 1–2 units of botulinum toxin at each site in the deep intradermal plane. The dose should not exceed 10–20 units per treatment session (Fig. 7.2).

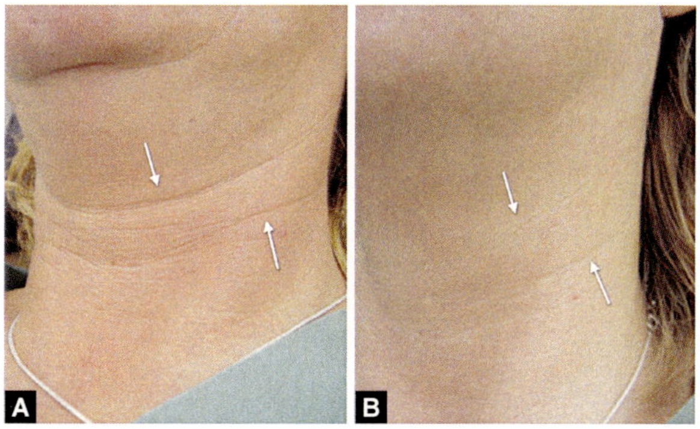

Figs 7.2A and B: (A) Before and (B) after—56 years/female—Correction of Nefertiti lines

3. *Platysmal bands:* Anterior platysmal bands become more visible while speaking, exercising or playing a musical instrument. Patient is asked to contract anterior neck by clenching teeth. It will exaggerate bands. Hold between thumb and index finger, insert into band and feel resistance. Inject 1–2 units into band perpendicularly at 1.0–1.5cm intervals from the jawline to the lower neck. Thinner bands respond to 5–10 units, while thicker bands respond to 10–15 units. Total dose of 20–30 units is delivered. Good patient selection is very important with good cervical skin elasticity and minimal fat descent (Fig. 7.3).
   Side-effects: Dysphagia, dystonia, weakness of muscles.

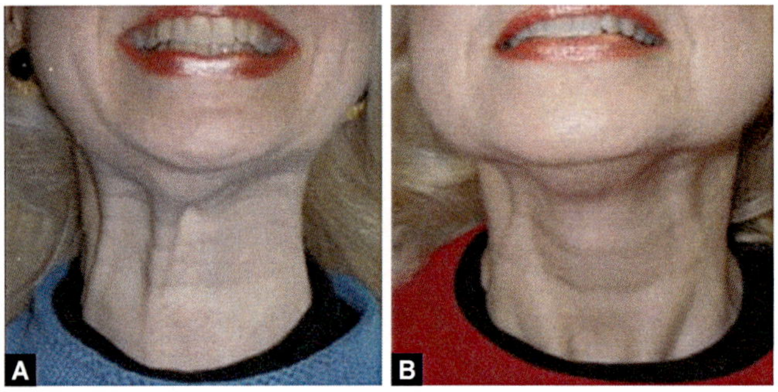

Figs 7.3A and B: (A) Before and (B) after—46 years/female—Correction of platysmal lines

4. *Mental crease/Popply chin:* Deep semilunar groove interposed between perioral area and prominence of chin is called mental crease. 2–5 units is injected into depressor anguli oris lower down close to its junction with inferior border of mandible (Fig. 7.4).

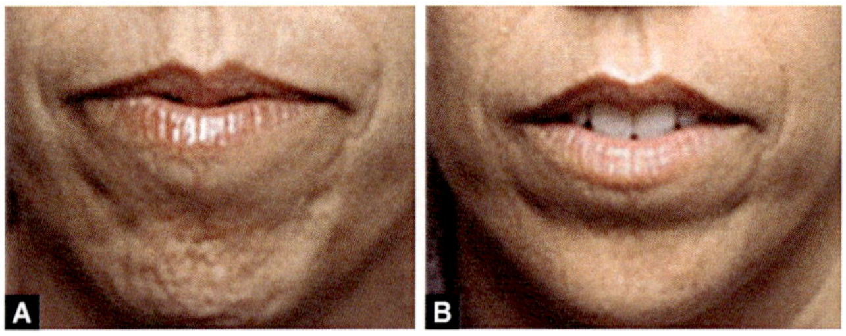

Figs 7.4A and B: (A) Before and (B) after—34 years/female—Correction of popply chin

5. *Bunny lines:* Contraction of muscular fibers of upper nasalis across the bony dorsum of nose cause bunny lines. Injection point should be anterior to the nasofacial groove on the lateral wall of the nose and well above angular vein to avoid affecting levator labii superioris alaque nasi (Fig. 7.5).

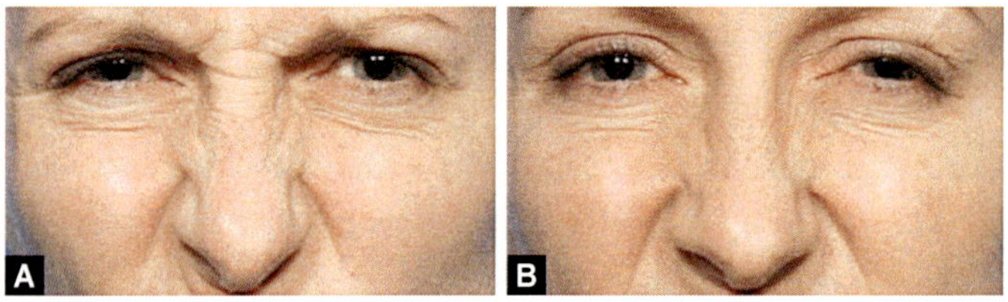

Figs 7.5A and B: (A) Before and (B) after—32 years/female—Correction of bunny lines

6. *Repeated nasal flare:* It is repeated dilatation of nostrils under social limitations. Injection of botulinum toxin in lateral nasalis fibers draped over lateral nasal ala will weaken its involuntary action (Fig. 7.6).

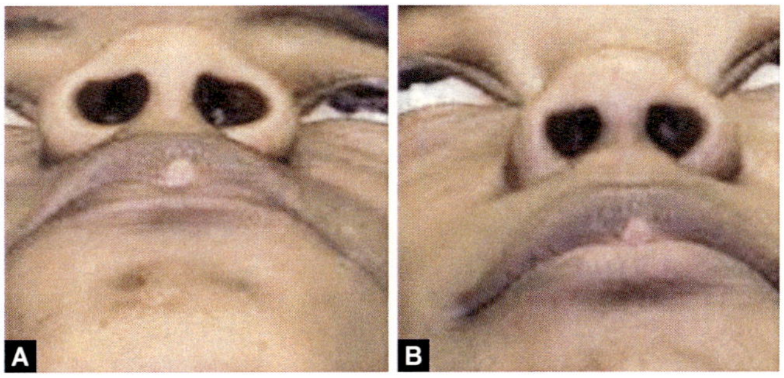

Figs 7.6A and B: (A) Before and (B) after—28 years/female—Correction of nasal flare

7. *Gummy smile:* It is an abnormally high retraction of the upper lip when a patient smiles. One unit of botulinum toxin on each levator labii complex in each nasofacial groove will relax the upper lips (Fig. 7.7).

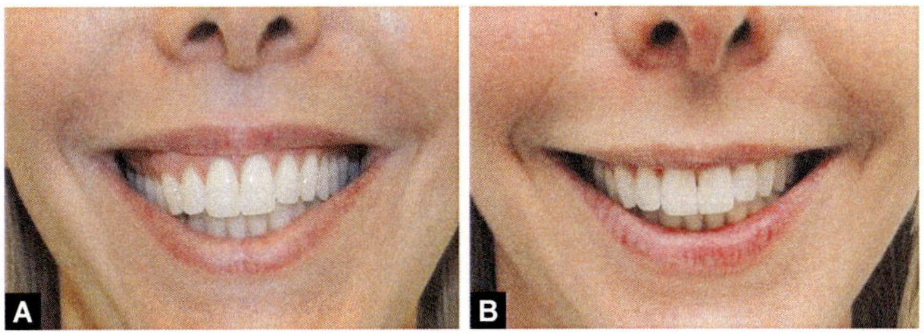

Figs 7.7A and B: (A) Before and (B) after—35 years/female—Correction of gummy smile

8. *Hypertrophic masseter:* One of the causes of square face is a hypertrophic masseter and the other is bony prominence of mandible. Masseter hypertrophy could be due to habitual chewing movements or teeth grinding (bruxism). Only superficial and medial head is injected. Draw an imaginary line between tragus of ear and corner of the mouth and inject only below this line. Ask the patient to clench teeth and mark the anterior and posterior border of masseter. Inject 1 cm inside anterior and posterior border of masseter. Inject 1cm above the angle of the mandible/jawline. Mark 3-5 points. Maximum dose of 15 units per side (Fig. 7.8).
   Side effects
   - Temporary pain/tenderness
   - Inability to chew hard/open the jaw
   - Asymmetry.

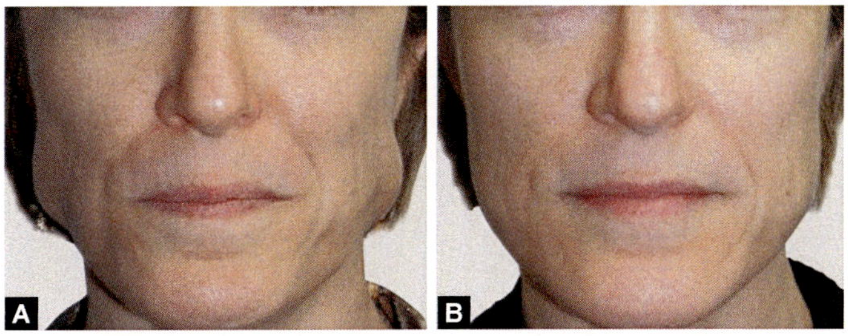

Figs 7.8A and B: (A) Before and (B) after—46 years/female—Correction of hypertrophic masseter

9. *Hyperhidrosis:* Done to reduce sweating in the axilla.The recommended dose is 50 units per axilla. The hyperhidrotic area to be injected should be defined using standard staining techniques, eg: Minor's iodine—Starch test. Using 30 gauge needle, 50 units of botulinum toxin is injected intradermally at a depth of 2mm. Inject 1-2 units per cm, at a angle of 45 degree to the skin surface with bevel side up to minimize leakage (Fig. 7.9).

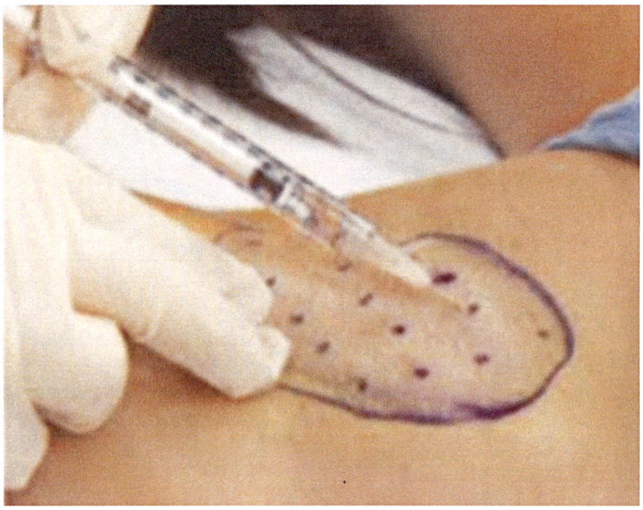

Fig. 7.9: Indicative diagram of hyperhidrosis injection points

FREQUENTLY ASKED QUESTIONS

What is botulinum toxin?

Botulinum toxin is a neurotoxin that temporarily relaxes muscle tissue. It has been used safely and extensively in medicine for over 10 years. It is one of the most popular cosmetic procedures.

Is botulinum toxin safe?

Absolutely, botulinum toxin has been safely used in medicine for over 10 years.

How does botulinum toxin reduce the signs of aging?

Minute amounts of botulinum toxin are injected into the appropriate muscles causing them to relax. This reduces or eliminates the appearance of wrinkles.

Are there any side effects?

The most common side effect of a botulinum toxin treatment is temporary bruising at the site of the injection. The bruising usually lasts only a few days and improves with time. In rare cases, the patient may temporarily experience a drooping eyelid. Some of these side effects can be minimized by choosing an experienced physician.

What are the treatments like?

Botulinum toxin injections are quick and painless. This is a 5–10 minute treatment where a very-fine needle is used to inject the botulinum toxin. This is truly a "lunchtime" procedure.

How long do the effects of the botulinum toxin last?

Botulinum toxin treatment usually last for 4–6 months.

Can botulinum toxin be used as part of my anti-aging strategy?

Yes, botulinum toxin can be used along with other anti-aging treatments, such as mesotherapy, wrinkle fillers or laser treatments.

What kind of results can I expect to see?

Proper injection of botulinum toxin is as much an art as it is a science. The goal of proper treatment is to diminish wrinkling and softening the lines.

8

CHAPTER

Dermal Fillers

INTRODUCTION

Dermal fillers are substances used in soft tissue augmentation to enhance or replace volume that is lost in any part of the skin or subcutaneous fat.

Fillers form an effective tool in rejuvenation, either as a stand-alone treatment or in combination with other procedures such as Laser resurfacing or botulinum toxin.

CLASSIFICATION

- Fillers can be classified based on different criteria:

Based on Longevity (Table 8.1)

Temporary

Temporary fillers are also referred to as nonpermanent fillers.

- They stay in the tissue is for less than 12 months and hence, they have the advantage of spontaneously disappearing if the patient is not satisfied with the results
- Similarly, an adverse event with such fillers is also a temporary one, as seen in the majority of the cases

TABLE 8.1: Types of fillers

Temporary (biodegradable) <1 year	*Semipermanent (biodegradable) 1–2 years*	*Permanent (nonbiodegradable) >2 tears*
Collagen	CaHA—Calcium hydroxylapatite	PMMA—Polymethylmethacrylate
Collagen—human	DEAE—Sephadex (Dextran)	PAAG—Polyacrylamide gel
Collagen—porcine	PLLA—Poly-L-lactic acid	Polyalkylimide
Hyaluronic acid—avian	PVA, Polyvinyl alcohol	LIS-Silicon (Polydimethylsiloxane oil)
Hyaluronic acid—bacterial	Chitosan HEMA, hydroxyethylmetacrylate Cultured human fibroblasts	

- They come in prefilled syringes having a particle size of 100–1250 microns and is most appropriate for mid-to-deep dermal injections
- Most of the fillers have a concentration of 20–24 mg/mL of hyaluronic acid

Some of the common temporary fillers available are described here:

Bovine collagen-based products

- Zyderm 1
- Zyderm 2
- Zyplast.

Human tissue-derived collagen

- Cosmoderm
- Cosmoplast.

Hyaluronic acid Fillers: A wide range of hyaluronic acid products is available with varying hyaluronic acid concentrations and cross-linking structure.

Semipermanent

These fillers undergo slow degradation with time over a period of 1–2 years. Side effects with semipermanent fillers are more common and longer lasting than temporary fillers.

Permanent

These are the fillers that remain for longer than two years in the tissue. Side effects with permanent fillers tend to be more permanent, and complication is the main issue with any permanent filler.

Based on Site of Placement (Fig. 8.1 and Tables 8.2 and 8.3)

Site of placement depends on particle size

- Superficial or fine line fillers ----100–150 microns
- Dermal ----150–280 microns
- Deep dermal ----280–500 microns
- Subdermal ----500–1250 microns
- Supraperiosteal ----1250–2000 microns

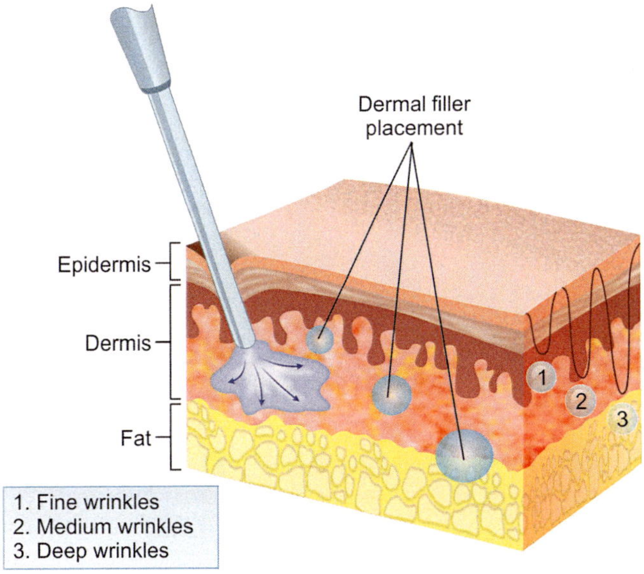

Fig. 8.1: Dermal filler placement

TABLE 8.2: Dermal filler chart

Material	*Site of placement*	*Longevity*	*Injection technique*	*FDA approval*
Artefill®	Reticular dermis	2 years	Layered, tunneling technique	Yes
Zydem® I × II Zyplast®	Dermis	2–4 months	Serial puncture, threading	Yes
Cosmodern®, Cosmoplast®	Dermis	2–4 months	Serial puncture, threading	Yes
Hyaluronic Acid				
Restylane®	Mid-dermis	6–8 months	Threading	Yes
Perlane®	Deep dermis	6–8 months	Threading and serial puncture	Yes
Hylaform®/Hylaform Plus®	Mid-dermis	4 months	Serial puncture and threading	Yes
Captique®	Mid-dermis	4 months	Serial puncture and threading	Yes
Juvederm®	Mid-dermis	4–8 months	Threading, serial puncture	Yes
Dermalive®	Mid-dermis	4–6 months	Threading, serial puncture	No
Autografts				
Autologous fat	Subcutis	> 1 year	Serial puncture Cross-hatching	Yes
Autologous fat	Mid-dermis Upper dermis	> 18 months	Threading	Yes
Synthetic materials				
Polytetrafluoroethylene	Subcutis	Permanent	Threading	Yes
Silicone	Deep dermis and subcutis	Permanent	Threading	Yes
Bioalcamid®	Subcutis	Permanent	Threading	No
Radiesse®	Deep dermis	9–18 months	Threading	Noncosmetic
Sculptra®	Deep dermis	1–2 Years	Threading	HIV lipoatrophy
Aquamid®	Subcutaneous	> 1 year	Threading	No

TABLE 8.3: Dermal filler characteristics

Dermal filler characteristic checklist Optimal characteristics-temporary fillers	
• Long duration/persistence	• No migration
• Performance promise	• Non-animal origin
• Painless	• Easy to inject
• Reasonable cost	• Easy to store
• Nontoxic	• Ease of learning how to inject
• Noninflammatory	• Minimal side effects
• Noncarcinogenic	• Biodegradable (in case of temporary and semipermanent fillers)

Based on Origin of Filler Material

Heterografts

1. Bovine collagen
   - Zyderm 1 and 2
   - Zyplast
   - Restoplast
   - Artecoll
2. Hyaluronic acid derivative implant
   - Restylane
   - Perlane
   - Juvederm
   - Revanesse
3. Porcine collagen
   - Permacol
   - Fibrel

Allografts: Human Derived Collagen

1. Dermalogen
2. Alloderm
3. Cosmoderm

Autograft

1. Autologous fat
2. Autologous collagen

Synthetic Material

1. Polytetrafluoroethylene
2. Silicone
3. Biopolymer 3
4. Bioplastique
5. Polyacrylamide

IDEAL DERMAL FILLER (FIG. 8.2)

Indications

- Facial lines (wrinkles, folds)
- Lip enhancement
- Facial deformities
- Depressed scars
  - Post-surgical
  - Traumatic
  - Acne and chickenpox scars
- Periocular melanoses, sunken eyes
- Dermatological diseases—angular cheilitis, scleroderma, AIDS lipoatrophy
- Breast, buttock augmentation.

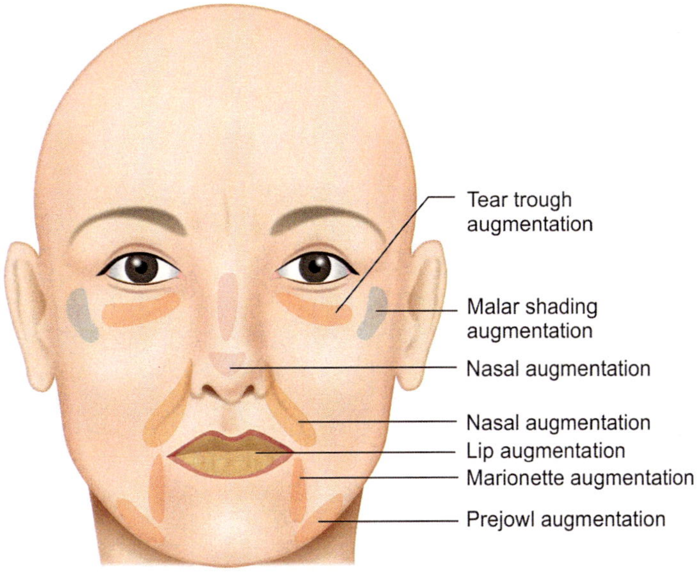

Fig. 8.2: Different areas on face needs to be corrected by filler

CONTRAINDICATIONS

- Positive skin test
- Patient with autoimmune diseases
- History of serious anaphylactic reaction in past
- Active local disease like acne
- Keloidal tendency
- Unrealistic expectations.

CONDITIONS REQUIRING CAUTION

- History of facial herpes simplex
- History of atopy (allergic reaction that becomes apparent in a sensitized person only minutes after contact)
- History of bleeding disorder or use of anticoagulants
- Current or long-term use of immunosuppressive therapy.

PREOPERATIVE PREPARATION

- History taking should include history of medications used, history of allergies, e.g., the chances of bruising might increase in a patient on anticoagulant therapy, aspirin or NSAIDS
- Clinical examination, particularly of the area being injected
- Skin test should be done if heterograft implants are used
- Counseling
- Preoperative photography is preferable
- Informed consent should be taken.

Skin Test

- It is done in two steps and 2 weeks prior to treatment
- Bovine collagen 0.1 mL and porcine collagen 0.05 mL (diluted in normal saline) is injected intradermally on the flexor aspect of forearm
- A positive skin test develops as early as 6–48 hours or 4 weeks after the test dose
- There is erythema, pruritis or prolonged induration that lasts for more than 4 days
- Inspite of negative skin test, there is a 1.2–6.3% chance of hypersensitivity, hence a second skin test after 4 weeks is advised
- If there is no sign of positivity after 2 weeks of second test, bovine/porcine collagen implants can be given with minimal risk of allergy.

INTRAOPERATIVE PROCEDURE

1. Surgical preparation of the part.
2. Topical anesthetics can be used 40 minutes to 1 hour before injection.
3. Local anesthesia required in upper lip augmentation and in uncooperative patient.
4. Patient is to be treated under proper lighting in semireclining or upright position for the gravity to maximize wrinkles.
5. All dermal fillers come with prefilled syringes and desired gauge needle (26–32 G) depending on the particle size. The needle should be screwed carefully on to the syringe to avoid waste of material.
6. The syringe should be levered over thumb of nonoperating hand for proper angle and depth of injection.
7. A 15 degree angle for superficial and 45 degree for deeper dermal implants are maintained.
8. Needle is inserted with bevelled surface facing upwards.
9. Blanching should be avoided.
10. The requisite depth of injection depends upon the nature of material used.
11. The material is injected in serial puncture, linear threading, fan or cross-hatching technique.
12. The defect fills up immediately.

13. Over correction is recommended only for lip augmentation.
14. Stop injection prior to withdrawal of needle to avoid unnecessary spillage.
15. Treated area is massaged lightly to mould the material appropriately and avoid lump formation.
16. Maximum of 2 mL of filler per treatment session is indicated.
17. Care should be taken to avoid injecting into a blood vessel.
18. If needle gets blocked, the pressure on the piston should not be increased rather injection should be stopped and needle replaced.
19. Repeat injection for correction should only be administered after 2–4 weeks when inflammation subsides totally.

INJECTION TECHNIQUES (FIGS 8.3A TO F)

1. *Linear threading techniques:* Full length of the needle is inserted into the defect and the implant is injected while pulling the needle slowly backwards so that the material is placed lengthwise in the wrinkle.
2. *Serial punture technique:* Multiple injections are placed serially along the length of the treated area so that it merges into a continuous line which lifts the wrinkle.
3. *Fan technique:* After injecting one line of implant by the linear-threading technique, the direction of the needle is changed and injected as before along a new line.
4. *Cross-hatching technique:* Cross-hatching technique is used at the periphery of the defect. Then the needle is withdrawn from the skin and inserted 5–10 mm adjacent to the first site of injection and procedure is repeated. This method is then carried out at right angles to the original line.

POST-PROCEDURE INSTRUCTIONS

- Avoid exposure to extreme cold or heat
- Avoid massaging treated areas for six hours
- Avoid strenuous physical activity for forty-eight hours
- Sleep with the head elevated for one night
- Pain medication can be taken if needed
- Resume skin care products, such as retinoids, alpha hydroxy acids two days after the procedure
- Chemical peels, laser treatment should be spaced out at least 2 weeks to avoid inflammation of injection site
- Repeat injections are spaced after 4–6 months or longer depending upon the longevity of the material, site of injection and the technique used.

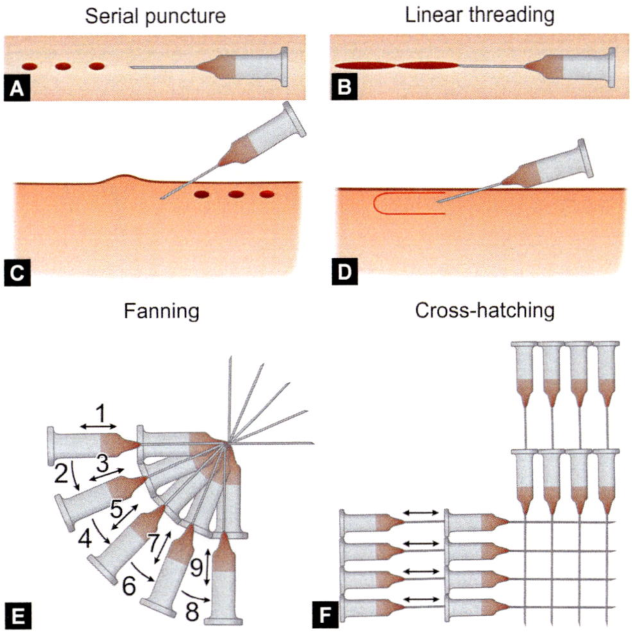

Figs 8.3A to F: Different techniques of injecting

COMBINATION TECHNIQUE

Combining two fillers of different particle size or other materials for enhanced cosmetic result:

1. Sandwich method: It is a layered technique using Perlane in deeper dermis and Restylane above it in mid or upper dermis.
2. Botulinum toxin and fillers: Botulinum toxin injected 1–2 weeks prior to dermal fillers gives a synergistic effect. Botox reduces the amount of implant for augmentation and also helps to increase the duration of the fillers in the treated area by reducing supposed muscle atrophy and prevent immediate microextrusion from injection sites by repetitive muscular action.

COMPLICATIONS

Immediate Complications

- Pain
- Bruising
- Erythema
- Asymmetry, bumpiness, lumpiness
- Anaphylaxis
- Edema
- Acneiform eruptions
- Infections—reactivation of herpes simplex.

Late Complications

- Inflammatory nodule
- Tyndall effect
- Allergic reactions
- Vascular occlusion
- Granulomas
- Implant migration
- Telangiectasia
- Lipoatrophy
- Hypertrophic scarring
- Sterile abscess.

ADVANTAGES OF DERMAL FILLERS

1. Instant results, no down time.
2. Easy technique compared to other procedures for scar or wrinkle correction, i.e. punch excision, punch graft replacement, etc.
3. Does not require special surgical expertise.
4. Simple OPD procedure.
5. Large area/multiple lesions covered at one sitting.

DISADVANTAGES OF DERMAL FILLERS

1. It is short lasting hence has to be repeated once in 6 months to a year.
2. Expensive treatment.
3. Chances of adverse reactions.

CONCLUSION (FIGS 8.4 TO 8.6)

- In a short span of time, fillers have come to play an important role in the nonsurgical management of ageing skin
- The technique is a safe, simple and effective modality, when used by a properly trained physician

- Proper knowledge of the anatomy of the area of injection, aesthetic sense and proper patient selection are essential
- Fillers can also be combined with other esthetic treatments such as Botox, Microdermabrasion, Peels, thread-lifts, and laser resurfacing
- As in all aesthetic techniques, proper patient counselling with respect to achievable results is important.

GENERAL FAQs FOR PATIENTS

Will I need a skin test?

Dermal filler is made of a natural, biocompatible substance that is identical to what's naturally found in the body. Because dermal filler does not contain any animal or human-derived components, there is virtually no risk of an allergic reaction. That means you do not need to undergo skin allergy testing prior to treatment. However, if you believe you are having an allergy to dermal filler, seek medical attention immediately.

Does it hurt?

Dermatologists use a variety of pain management techniques during treatment to ensure patient comfort. Topical anesthetic cream application being the most commonly used technique to numb the area of injection, making the procedure less painful.

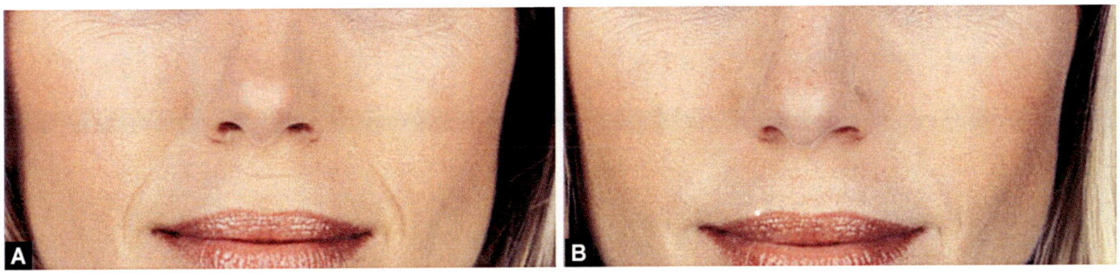

Figs 8.4A and B: (A) Before and (B) after—38 years/female—Soften nasolabial folds

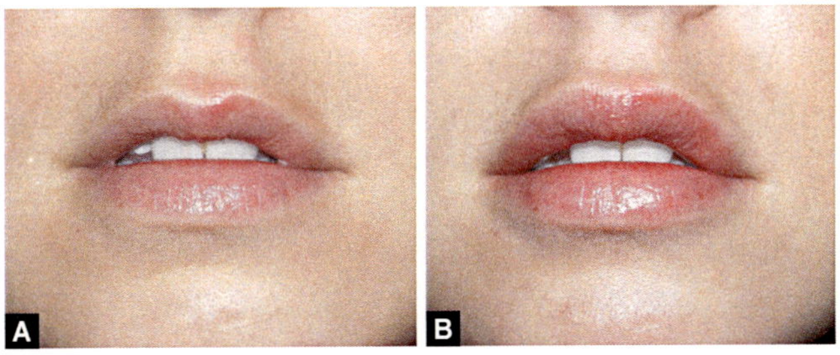

Figs 8.5A and B: (A) Before and (B) after 36 years/female—Lip enhancement

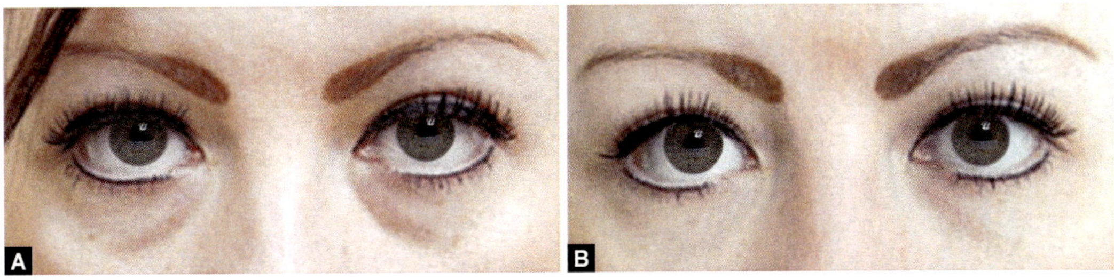

Figs 8.6A and B: (A) Before and (B) after 38 years/female—Tear trough filler

Are there any side effects?

There have been very few side effects reported in clinical trials and actual usage. However, you may experience some common injection-related reactions, such as mild irritation, edema, swelling, itching, discoloration, or tenderness at the injection site. These conditions typically resolve themselves within one to two days.

What if the patient is on any medication?

Patients may need to refrain from taking some medications and supplements for a few days prior to treatment. Please take a detailed history of the patient and informed consent before doing the procedure.

How soon can I expect results?

You will see results immediately after treatment. Semipermanent dermal filler continues to deliver results over time as it stimulates your body to produce new collagen. Results may last up to a year or more in many patients, which may result in fewer visits for retreatment.

How quickly can I return to my normal activities?

Most patients experience little to no downtime and return to normal activities almost immediately after treatment. A maximum of 24 hours after treatment, most of the swelling and redness will have subsided.

How long will the results last?

Treatment results last up to a year or more for many patients. Individual results may vary, depending on age, skin type, lifestyle, and metabolic rate, so be sure to discuss patient expectations.

How many treatments are required?

Many patients will achieve their desired result after just one treatment. To ensure satisfaction, schedule a follow-up visit, where a touchup treatment might be recommended.

Are there different types of fillers?

The standard has long been hyaluronic acid fillers. Recently newer fillers such as semipermanent or permanent have become available. Each filler has its own benefits. Some of the fillers are being used "off label". This means that the filler has been FDA approved for use in another area. This is similar to the way Botox® and other medications are used.

Are there disadvantages of longer lasting fillers?

Yes, the more permanent fillers make it difficult to make corrections. To ensure good results shorter acting filler should be tried first. If you are happy with the results, a longer lasting filler can be used at a later date.

Are there any side effects?

Possible side effects vary from filler to filler.

9

CHAPTER

Thread Lift

WHAT IS THREAD LIFT?

A cosmetic procedure that lifts and realigns sagging tissue while adding definition to facial contours by using absorbable 'threads'.

This procedure helps to reposition sagging cheeks, lift eyebrows, correct marionette lines, support the neck and improve facial features.

INDICATIONS

- Lift and add volume to sagging cheeks
- Elevate sagging brows
- Correct marionette lines and nasolabial folds
- Support and revitalize the neck area
- Correct asymmetry of the brow and face
- Revitalize and lift the jowl area.

CLIENT SELECTION

- Suitable candidates for a thread lift procedure are those who are experiencing mild to moderate sagging of facial tissues, usually those in their forties to late fifties
- These clients do not want or are not ready for surgery but want something more than what cosmetic injectable or skin resurfacing/skin tightening procedures can offer.

Suitable candidate for thread lift:

- Moderate sagging and laxity of the skin in the cheeks, eyebrows, eyes, jowls and neck
- Effects of a previous face-lift or neck-lift are wearing off
- Younger clients with cheek and brow sagging caused by weakened tissue (ptosis)
- Clients having realistic expectations.

Unsuitable candidates for thread-lift surgery include:
- Clients with very thin, fragile skin associated with advance facial aging
- Clients with heavy jowls and excess skin, which require surgical removal
- Clients who do not have realistic expectations and those with any medical contraindications.

BENEFITS OF THREAD LIFT (FIG. 9.1)

- Giving your face a subtle and more natural-looking lift
- Relatively no downtime compared to other cosmetic procedures
- Lower cost as compared to a surgical facelift
- Stimulates collagen production and therefore, helps in skin rejuvenation.

TYPES OF THREAD USED

Simple Thread (Fig. 9.2)

The thread used in this procedure is absorbable monofilament thread, USP size 5-0~7-0 (PDO: Polydioxanone), half-folded attached with size 25~31 G needle (Table 9.1). It is injected into the skin and the thread will become V-shaped and stay there.

TABLE 9.1: Threads and needle size chart

Size	*Length*
31 G	30 mm
29 G	40 mm 50 mm
27 G	60 mm
25 G	90 mm

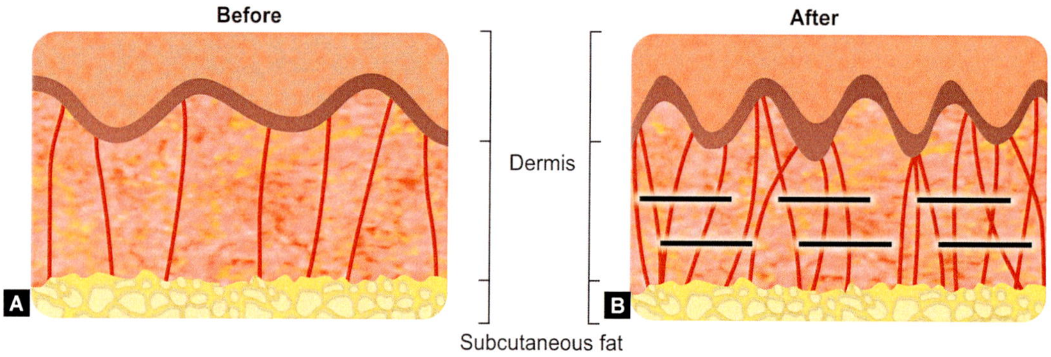

Figs 9.1A and B: Collagen building after threads

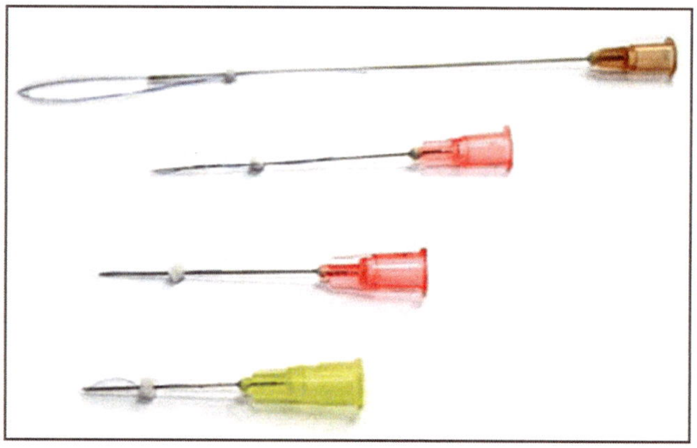

Fig. 9.2: Threads needles

Cogged or Barbed Thread (Fig. 9.3)

These are essentially mono threads with barbs to hook to the underside of the skin. The barbs form a support structure that lifts the sagging tissue. Unlike mono threads, cog threads do not need anchoring points. Collagen formation can also occur around the threads and their barbs. Cog threads are most effective for jawline lifting and body contouring.

They are divided into different categories depending on the direction of their cogs/barbs (Fig. 9.4D):

1. Convergent or divergent threads, depending on whether the cogs are orientated towards each other or in opposite directions from each other from the middle.
2. Unidirectional or bidirectional threads, depending on whether the cogs are orientated in only one direction, or in opposite directions.
3. These threads are made of a non-absorbable monofilament material (a single strand of fiber) called polypropylene, which has been used for surgical sutures (stitches) for many years. They are designed with bidirectional cogs or barbs that go outwards from the middle of the thread and point inwards towards the middle (convergent), so that as they are inserted under the skin the cogs anchor and hold the lift.

Mono threads are smooth threads without barbs. Many of these thread type are placed into the face in a mesh-like fashion for skin tightening effect. Skin tightening usually improves after collagen starts forming around the threads. The treatment areas are often neck lines, sagging neck, forehead and under the eyes. Approximately—10–20 mono threads are usually inserted for each treatment area. In order to sustain a lift, the threads are attached to an "anchoring point" of the scalp or face. Mono threads tighten the skin but without significant lifting; therefore they have to be used with cog threads for an overall improvement in face tightening and rejuvenation (Fig. 9.4A).

Screw threads can come in the form of one or two threads intertwined together around the inserting needle. Screw thread has a great effect on giving volume effect on sunken area of the skin. Multi Screw—when intertwining two threads are used—has stronger effect over screw thread. Screw threads are usually used for general face-lifting (Fig. 9.4C).

There are many variations like mono screw thread, Tornado thread (Fig. 9.5), Tornado screw thread, etc. All being combinations of the above mentioned types.

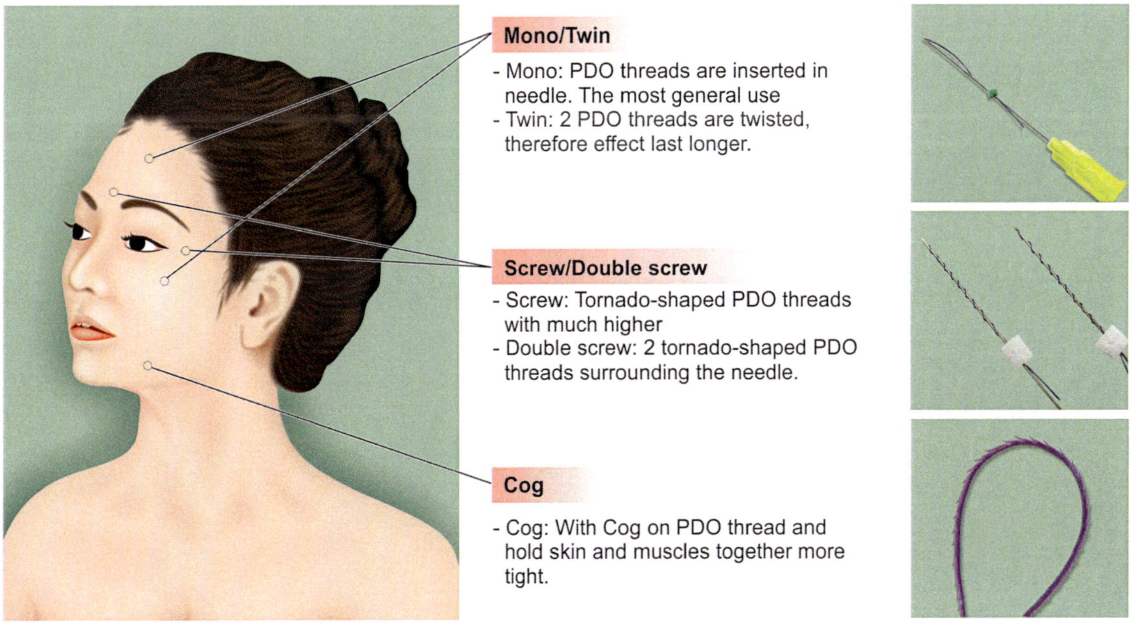

Fig. 9.3: Types of threads

PROCEDURE

- Procedure takes place under topical anesthesia (with lidocaine cream or nerve blocking with injectable lidocaine) for at least 45 minutes
- After topical anesthesia, the thread lift needles are inserted in the dermis of the area you need to treat
- After inserting the needle just pull back the needle slowly and the thread will be left behind
- The procedure takes approximately 30 minutes per area. The amount of the threads depends on the area to be treated
- No incisions or stitches are required, and no scars are produced. There is either no surgical scar or wound. However, you may see a few bruises, which can fade overtime within a few days
- You will see immediate improvement (20–30%) after the application, with remarkable improvement after 2–3 weeks. The best results will be remarkable after 2 months. PDO lifting threads will be absorbed in 6 months and results lasts up to 12–18 months.

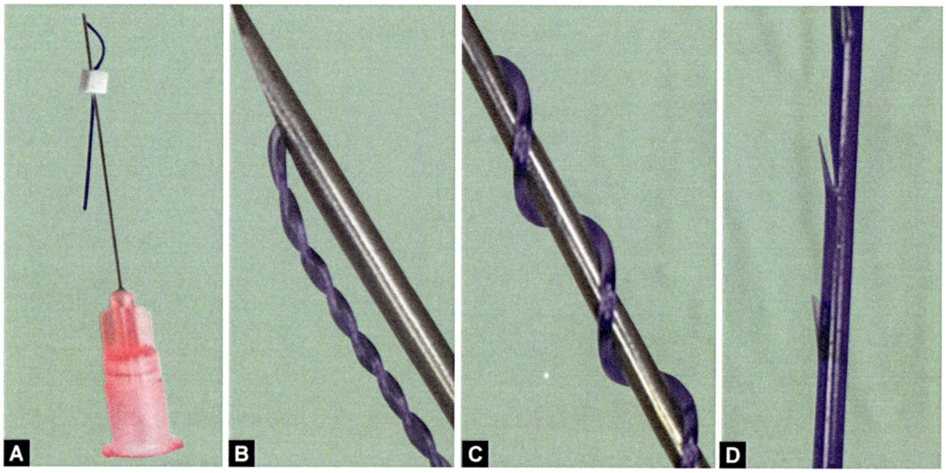

Figs 9.4A to D: (A) Normal thread; (B) Tomado thread; (C) Screw thread; (D) Cogged thread

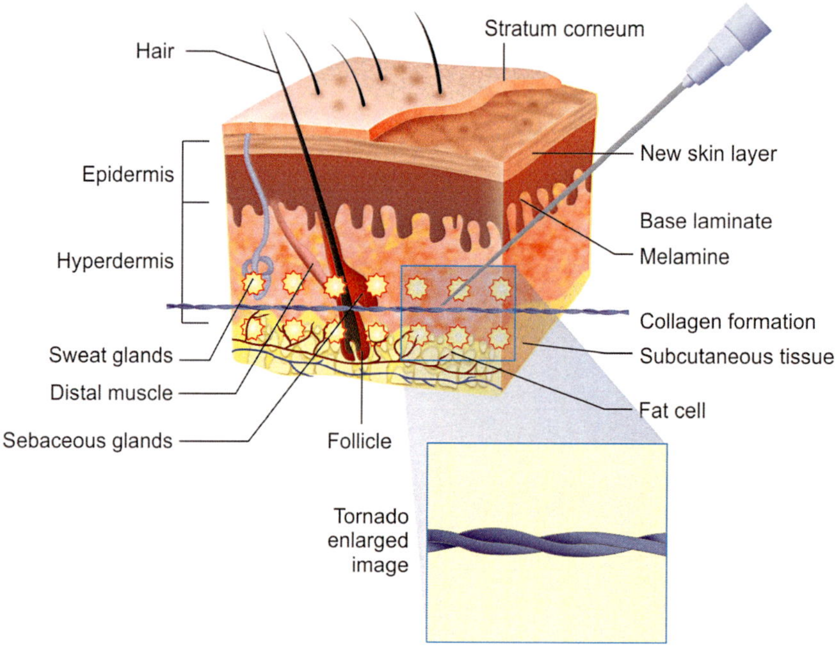

Fig. 9.5: Placement of Tornodo thread

Recommendations after Treatment

- To limit facial activity
- To avoid heavy exercises
- To avoid temperature fluctuations
- Avoid any other cosmetic procedure for 3 weeks.

Recovery

- Postprocedure you may experience some slight bruising and swelling, which usually settles in a few days
- Oral painkillers and prophylactic antibiotics are prescribed as well. Recovery is generally quick, with most clients returning to work on the same or next day
- Advice clients to avoid eating hard food
- Normal physical activities may be resumed three days after the thread procedure. Bruising can be covered up with medical make up
- Avoid rubbing or contorting your face for three weeks after thread lift surgery
- Avoid any other procedures on the skin for at least 3 weeks.

Results (Figs 9.6 to 9.9)

- Results of thread lift are seen after 1 to 3 months after the procedure.
- The results last from 12 to 18 months in younger clients.

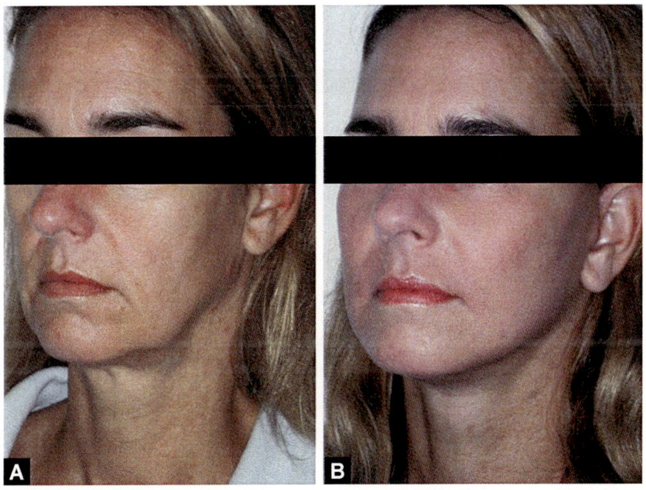

Figs 9.6A and B: (A) Before and (B) after—38 years/female—Lower jowls and neck

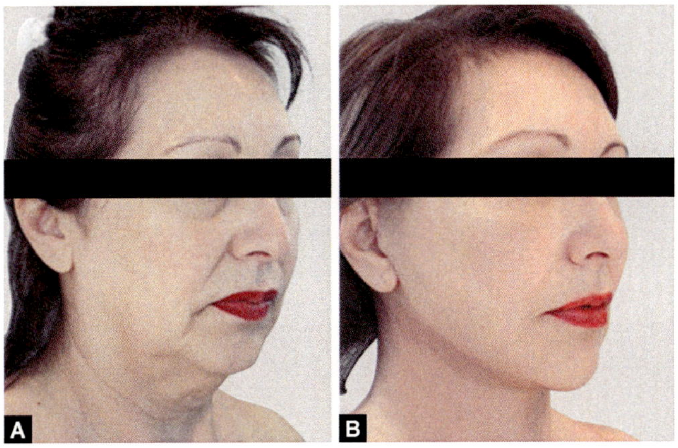

Figs 9.7A and B: (A) Before and (B) after—46 years/female—Lower jowls and neck

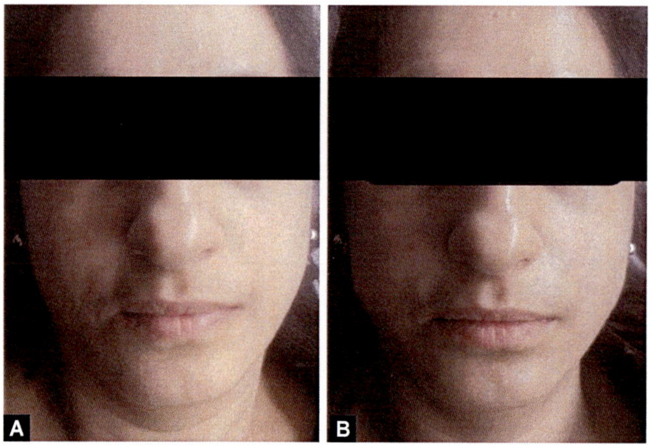

Figs 9.8A and B: (A) Before and (B) after—44 years/female—Cheek and neck

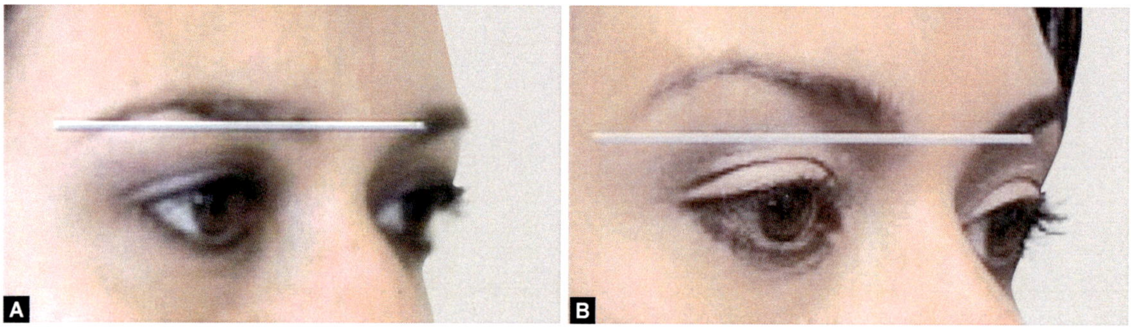

Figs 9.9A and B: (A) Before and (B) after—32 years/female—Brow lift

COMPLICATION

Bruising and swelling may occur immediately after the procedure: This is natural, and you can expect it to resolve on its own. Severe swelling should be reported to your doctor immediately as this could be due to an infection.

Infections: If there is an infection in the treated area, prescribe antibiotics to the patients.

Visible threads: In clients with thin skin, the threads may become visible underneath the skin soon after the procedure. This is temporary and will improve once the thread starts dissolving. Sometimes, clients may feel the thread has come out from where it was inserted, in that case just ask the client to cut the protruding thread. This is common in patients with more skin laxity.

Numbness or lack of sensitivity: These sensations will usually disappear within weeks but contact your doctor if they persist.

CONTRAINDICATIONS

Absolute Contraindication

- Skin infection and inflammation
- During pregnancy and lactation
- On anticoagulant medication
- Clients who have blood-related diseases (hemophilia)
- Keloidal tendency
- Uncontrolled diabetes mellitus
- Autoimmune diseases.

Relative Contraindication

- When sagging is serious and deep (over 70 years)
- Diabetes mellitus
- Any ongoing major illness.

GENERAL FAQ`S FOR PATIENTS

What is a thread lift?

A thread lift is a type of face lift that is often referred to as the "lunch hour lift". This is due to its simplicity and the time it takes to carry out the procedure. Fine threads are inserted and advanced along pre-marked contours. These threads have fine filaments that become fixed to the tissue and are then gently smoothed down. Your body then starts to produce new bundles of collagen which surround each filament and this in turn creates a subtle yet effective lift. The results differ for each person, but gives a very natural rejuvenated and refreshed look. There is no scarring and recovery time is a lot less than those associated with traditional surgery.

What areas can be treated with a thread lift?

The thread lift can be used to enhance and improve the appearance of a sagging neck, sagging cheeks and jowls and droopy eyebrows. You can personalize your surgery to suit your exact needs and your doctor will also make recommendations for improvements. The procedure can be tailored to suit your exact needs to ensure you are totally happy with the results.

What are the advantages of a thread lift?

The great thing about a thread lift is that it offers quick recovery together with excellent results. This procedure requires a minimum amount of invasive surgery and leaves no scarring. Local anesthetic is all that is required and there is no hospital stay required. Another good factor about the thread lift is that it is much more affordable than a regular face lift and the results are long lasting. If you are looking for a quick and effective solution to a range of aging problems then a thread lift is the perfect solution.

Who is a thread lift suited for?

A thread lift is more suited to men and women between the ages of 40 and 60. The procedure is most effective on skin that has minimal sagging and offers the best results for cheeks, jowls, brows and the neck area. If you are looking for results that are more effective and long lasting than Botox and other fillers, then a thread lift is the ideal choice. If you are put off by traditional surgery then a thread lift is great as it is minimally invasive and can be carried out under local anesthetic.

What are the risks?

Thread lifts can cause minor side effects such as infection, bruising, swelling, tenderness, numbness and slight asymmetry. All side effects should be explained in detail to you before the procedure is booked. Any side effects should disappear within a few days.

How long does a thread lift take?

A typical thread lift takes as little as one hour to perform, but the length will depend on the number of filaments the doctor uses and the areas being treated.

What happens after the procedure?

Once the procedure is complete you will be provided with aftercare instructions to follow. These will help to relieve any discomfort and help to speed up the process of healing. For the first 24–48 hours, you can use ice compresses to deal with any swelling and help to alleviate discomfort. Most patients experience some mild swelling and bruises, but these are usually quick to settle. Recovery times are usually less than one week although strenuous exercise should be avoided for between 2 and 3 weeks.

How long do the results last?

A thread lift's lasting power depends on the age of the patient at the time of procedure and how much sagging the thread lift has corrected. It should be noted that sagging will return over time, but many doctors report that the results last for anything between 12 to 18 months. To extend the results, it is possible to have additional filaments inserted and your doctor can advise you when this is required.

10

CHAPTER

Glutathione

INTRODUCTION

Glutathione is an antioxidant primarily made of 3 amino acids namely cystine, glycine, and glutamic acid (Fig. 10.1). It is the body's own antioxidant discovered in 1889. It is safe for everyone, no matter the age. It is considered to be the most powerful, most versatile and most important part of the body's self-generated antioxidants. It is found in almost all living cells. The liver, spleen, kidneys, pancreas, the lens and cornea, have the highest concentrations in the body. It is a powerful antioxidant and thus neutralizes free radicals and prevents their formation. It has an important role in immune function via white blood cell production and is one of the most potent anti-viral agents known. It is one of the strongest anti-cancer agents manufactured by the body. It is produced by the liver to detoxify toxins including formaldehyde, acetaminophen, benzopyrene, and many other compounds. It is an antioxidant necessary for the protection of proteins, it is involved in nucleic acid synthesis and plays a role in DNA repair. It maintains the cellular redox potential and protects the integrity of red blood cells. Glutathione is involved in maintaining normal brain function. It is listed in the united state food and drug administration (USFDAs) generally recognized as safe (GRAS) list of safe food supplements.

SOURCES: DIRECT SOURCES

Plant Sources (Fig. 10.2)

Glutathione is found in a variety of foods, particularly fruits, vegetables, and meats. Foods rich in glutathione include asparagus, spinach, garlic, avocado, squash, zucchini, potatoes, melons, grapefruit, strawberries, and peaches. Some foods contain other compounds which trigger the body's production of glutathione.

In order to receive the most glutathione from fruits and vegetables, it is important to consume them fresh, not cooked or processed. Cooking and processing will decrease the bioavailability of glutathione in these foods. In addition, glutathione levels vary widely among fruits and vegetables due to environmental factors and the plant's phase of development.

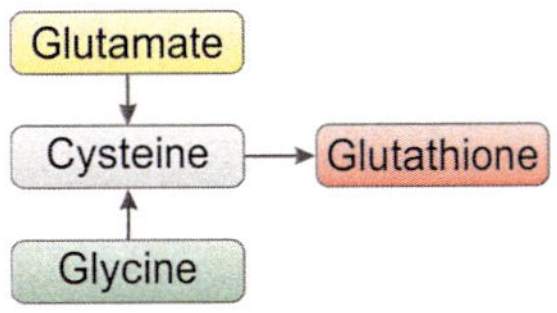

Fig. 10.1: Amino acids in glutathione

Animal Sources (Fig. 10.3)

Dietary glutathione is found in high amounts in fresh, uncooked meats and in moderate amounts in dairy products and eggs. These foods are high in whey protein containing alpha-lactalbumin which is rich in sulfur-containing amino acids. These products optimize the use of glutathione within the body. Cooking and prolonged storage reduces glutathione content of these foods. However, the glutathione content of these foods is high enough that consuming these products after cooking and processing provides the body with sufficient sources of glutathione.

Indirect Sources (Fig. 10.4)

- Selenium is an important co-factor for the enzyme form of glutathione. Selenium is necessary for formation of glutathione containing enzymes. For that reason, consuming foods rich in selenium will promote the production of glutathione. These foods include cereals, oats, Brazil nuts, walnuts, legumes, tuna, beef, poultry, cheese, eggs.
  Alpha lipoic acid, or ALA, promotes the synthesis of glutathione within the body, thereby increasing glutathione levels. Foods rich in alpha lipoic acid include: spinach, tomatoes, peas, Brussels sprouts, rice bran and mayonnaise. Many of these foods are naturally high in glutathione. Eating these foods increases the bioavailability of this important antioxidant.

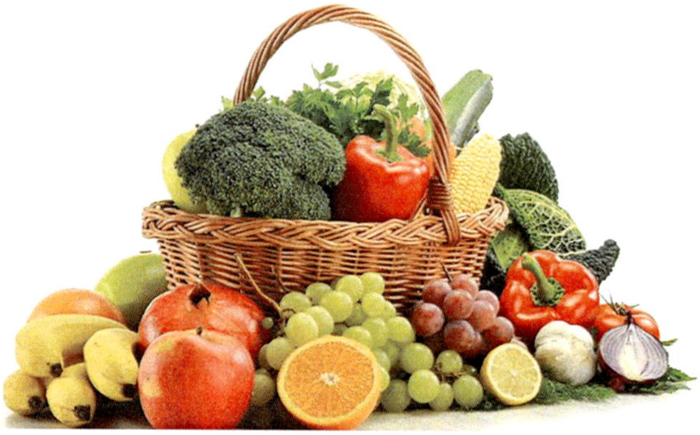

Fig. 10.2: Plant sources

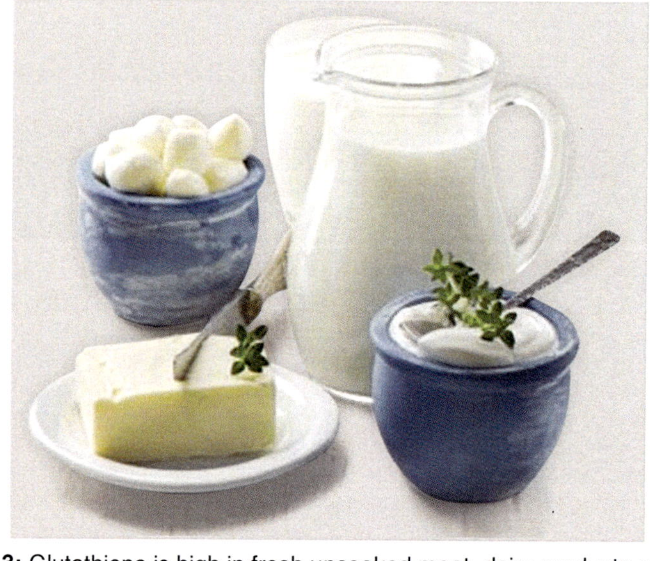

Fig. 10.3: Glutathione is high in fresh uncooked meat, dairy products and eggs

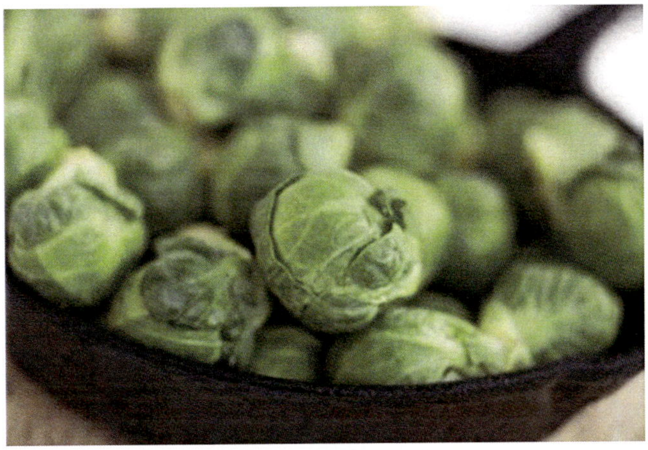

Fig. 10.4: Foods with selenium or alpha-lipoid acid

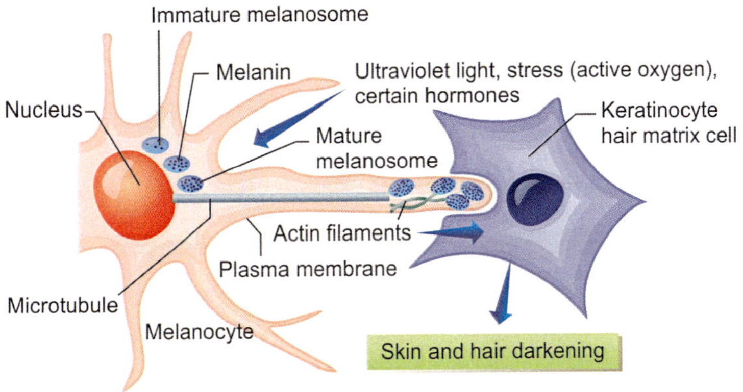

Fig. 10.5: Production on melanin. When melanocytes are activated by ultraviolet light, etc., melanin (schematically shown as granules) is formed around the nucleus and stored in small organelles known as melanosomes. Melanosomes are transported along microtubules and actin filaments to the cell periophery. Subsequently, melanosomes bind to the plasma membrane and transfers melanosomes to keratinocytes and hair matrix cells, resulting in skin and hair blackening

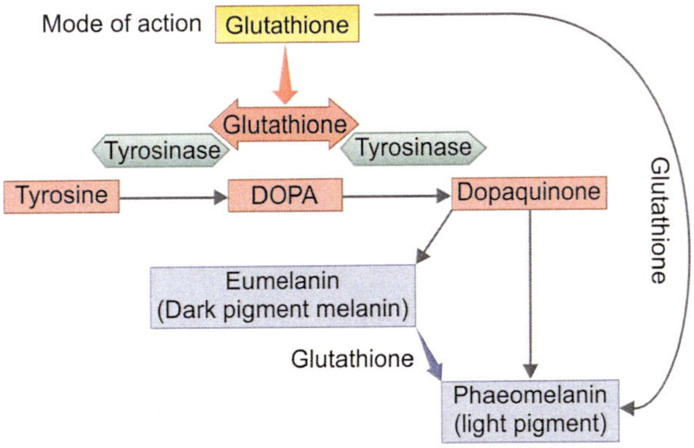

Fig. 10.6: Glutathione—mode of action

MECHANISM OF ACTION (FIGS 10.5 AND 10.6)

- Mediating the switch mechanism from eumelanogenesis (brown) to pheomelanogenesis (red-yellow)
- Its antioxidant properties help to neutralize the peroxides and free radicals which induce melanin synthesis and modulates the capabilities of melanocytotoxic agents in depigmentation and whitening.

FREE RADICALS (FIGS 10.7 TO 10.9)

- Small, diffusible molecules that differ from most biological molecules in that they have an unpaired electron.
- Free radicals tend to be reactive and can participate in chain reactions in which a single free radical initiation event can be propagated to damage multiple molecules.
- Once formed they react with other molecules, damaging the main constituents of cells.

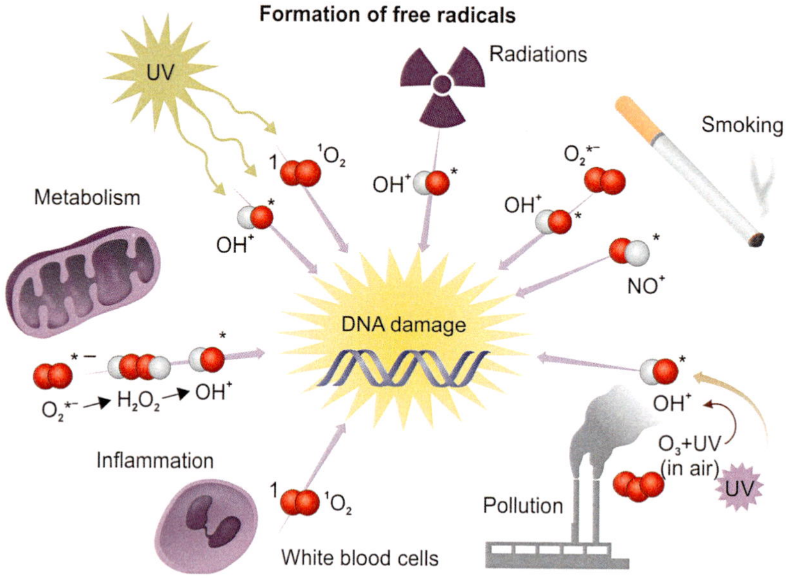

Fig. 10.7: Formation of free radicals

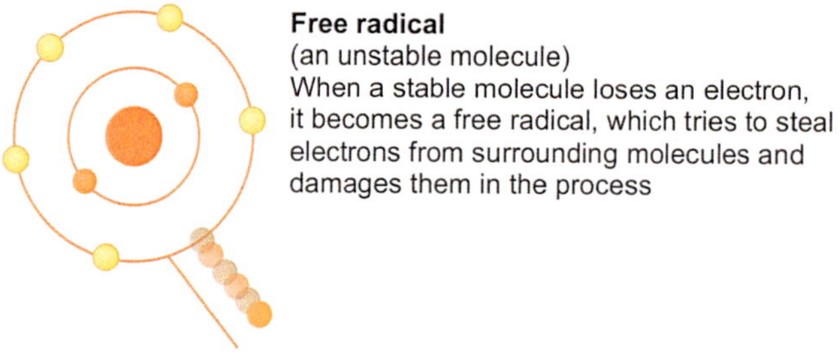

Fig. 10.8: What is free radical

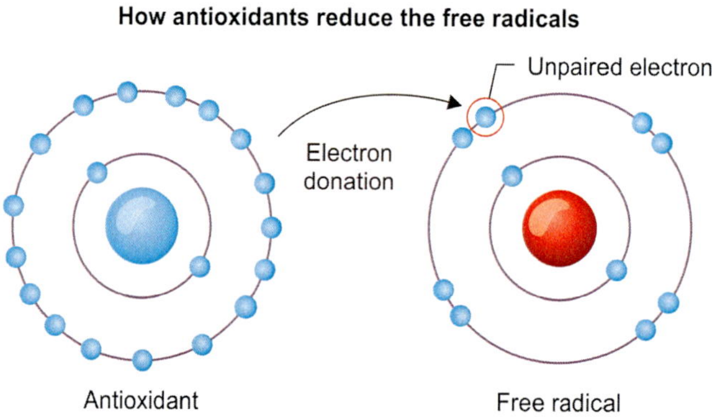

Fig. 10.9: Neutralization of free radicals

ROUTES OF ADMINISTRATION

- Oral
- Intravenous
- Sublingual
- Inhalation
- Topical.

INDICATIONS

- Fatty liver
- Treating or preventing alcoholism
- Cataracts
- Glaucoma
- Preventing aging
- Asthma
- Cancer
- Heart disease
- High cholesterol levels
- AIDS
- Chronic fatigue syndrome
- Memory loss
- Alzheimer's disease
- Osteoarthritis
- Parkinson's disease.

Other Conditions

- Reducing side effects of chemotherapy treatments for cancer
- Treating Parkinson's disease
- Diabetes
- Anemia in people on hemodialysis
- "Hardening of the arteries" (atherosclerosis)
- Infertility in men
- Other conditions.

CONTRAINDICATIONS

- Never use for people under chemotherapy. It may decrease the potency of anti-cancer drugs
- Not advised for people with chronic kidney failure and liver problem because it may cause digestive complications such as severe pain and persistent diarrhea
- Do not use during pregnancy and breastfeeding
- May worsen asthmatic episodes, thus it is not recommend for asthmatic individuals.

DRUG INTERACTION

- Vitamin K3, vitamin B_{12}, calcium pantothenate, orotic acid, antihistamines, sulfanilamide and tetracycline can affect the bioavailability of glutathione.

SIDE EFFECTS

- It can cause simple symptoms such as abdominal pain and loose bowel movement, and serious complications like renal injury, toxic epidermal necrolysis (TEN) and Steven Johnson syndrome (SJS)
- Oral glutathione has been found to induce hypersensitivity reactions, characterized by maculopapular and urticarial form of rashes, and even zinc deficiency, upon long term use
- Nebulized forms of glutathione have been found to assist in sulfite formation. These sulfites consequently cause difficulty of breathing, hence are contraindicated to some patients with asthma
- Thus, one should first weigh the pros and cons of glutathione use before intake. Furthermore, it would be of help if an expert physician be consulted prior glutathione consumption.

BENEFITS OF GLUTATHIONE

- Glutathione works from the inside to repair and nourish skin
- Helps to lighten your total body
- Gives skin a radiant glow
- Helps to improve skin hyper pigmentation
- Helps improve dark circles
- Helps controls acne and helps to prevents acne marks
- Helps to defy the aging process.

GLUTATHIONE IN SKIN LIGHTENING

- Glutathione is effective in skin lightening if taken it in a higher dose. The suggested dose of glutathione is 20–40 mg per kg body weight. For better results, one should quit smoking, liquor and sun exposure
- Recommended dose of vitamin C is twice the dose of reduced glutathione when given orally
- Results are usually visualized after 3–4 months of treatment

Duration of Intake for Skin Whitening (Fig. 10.10)

- *Medium brown:* 1–3 months
- *Dark brown:* 3–6 months
- *Very dark skin:* 6–12 months
- *Black skin:* At least 2 years or even more

Once a person has his/her desired skin color, the maintenance dose is required.

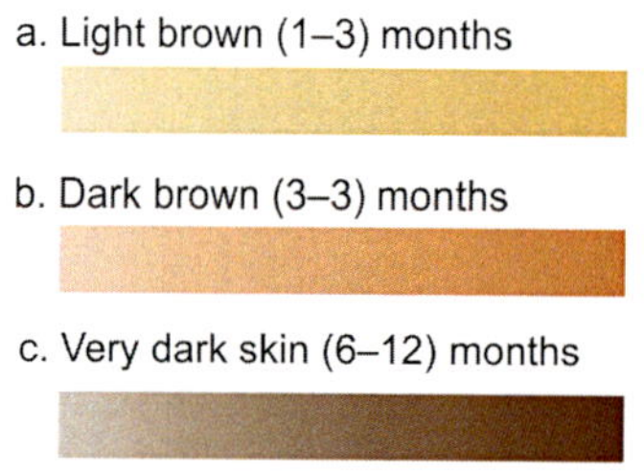

Fig. 10.10: Skin lightening chart

PRE- AND POST-PICTURES (FIGS 10.11 TO 10.13)

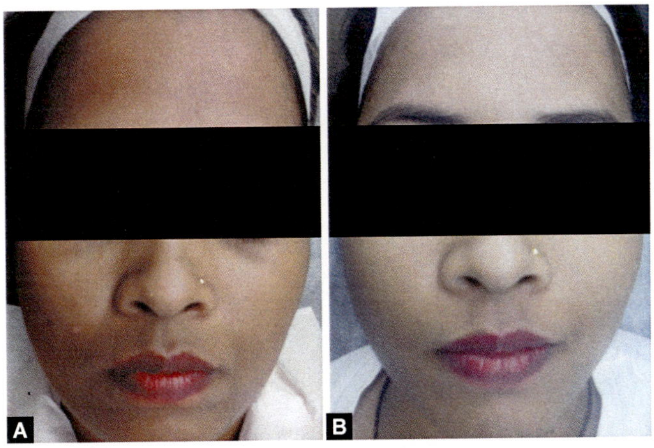

Figs 10.11A and B: (A) Before and (B) after—28 years/female—after 3 months

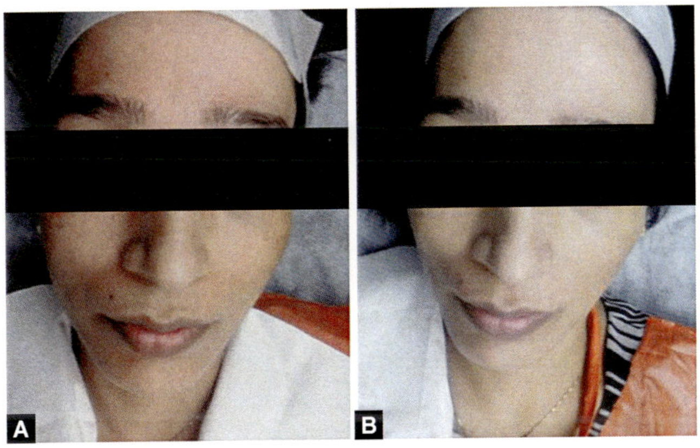

Figs 10.12A and B: (A) Before and (B) after—36 years/female—after 3 months

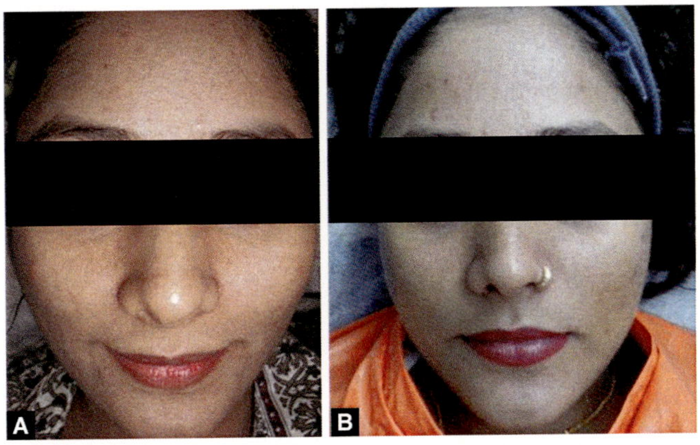

Figs 10.13A and B: (A) Before and (B) after—32 years/female—after 3 months

FAQS FOR PATIENTS

How long before I see the results?

Average 3–4 months are required to see optimum results. However, this may vary. Results have been documented as early as 3–4 weeks.

Why is it that some people see the results early and others took long before they can see it?

Metabolism and absorption varies from one individual to another. Weight is another factor affecting the absorption.

What makes L-glutathione different compared to other whitening pills/capsules?

Unlike any other whitening pills/capsules, glutathione is an anti oxidant, anti aging immune booster and detoxifier. There are no harmful effects on the body and is also recommended by doctors for people with liver problems and other conditions

Is it ok to continue your regular skin regimen such as applying of creams, lotions, gels while taking glutathione?

Yes, it is ok. These products can also help you enhance the results topically. Always consult your physician before application.

Tender Skin Cosmetology Academy

The number of professionally trained practitioners of aesthetic medicine/beauty care is far lower than required to serve the community.

Professionals wishing to practice cosmetic medicine hail from the medical community of physicians, dermatologists, plastic surgeons and from other allied and non-medical fields that include laser technicians, cosmetologists, beauticians, etc.

In most cosmetic clinics or similar set-ups, highly specialized procedures are being administered by non-medical staff instead of trained physicians, which may not have received adequate training and not have the skills to carry out these sensitive medical procedures.

Tender Skin International (TSI) Academy was started to fill the need—gap in the market for trained professionals in this booming beauty care industry and has also empowered over 500 students since it started in 2010. Our education and training center, provides technical training not only to students wishing to take up cosmetology as a career but also imparts training to professionals in the field wishing to up-grade their skills.

OUR STUDENT ENDORSEMENTS

STUDENT TESTIMONIALS

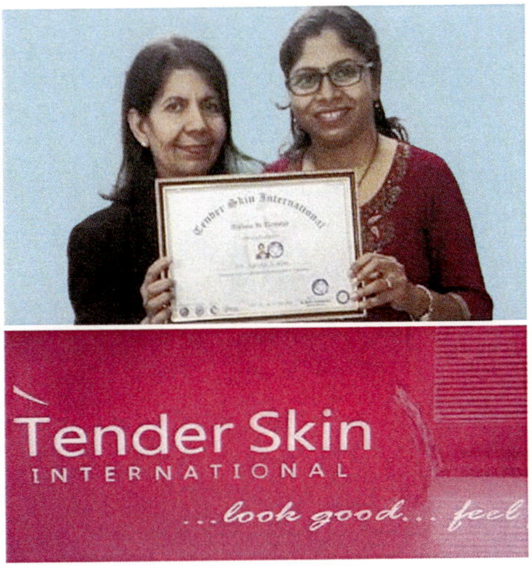

"Doing trichology and selected curriculum of Basic and Advanced Cosmetology from Tender Skin International Academy has given me tremendous confidence. I have learnt lots of procedures, done many of them personally which definitely is going to help me in my private practice. All the staff at TSI was extremely supportive. Your co-operation will always be appreciated. Looking forward in doing more courses from your academy. Thanks a lot."

—Dr Varsha S, Nashik

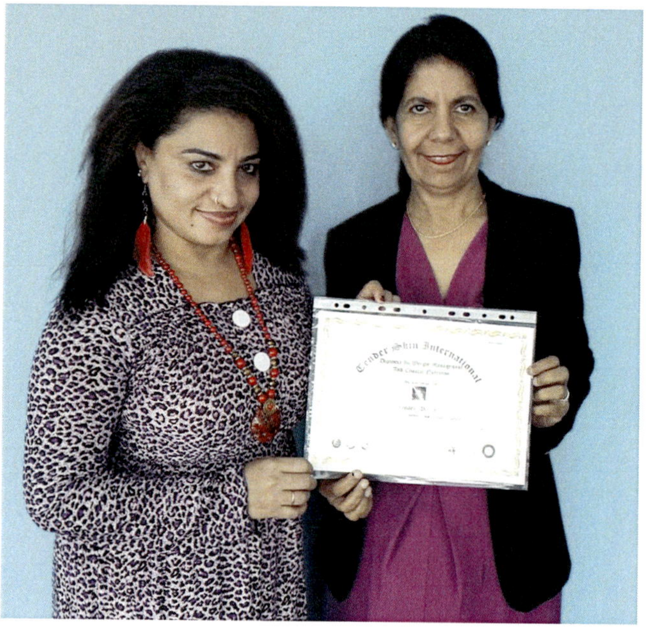

I took "Advanced Diploma in Cosmetology" from their institution and I can say it is one of the best courses which enabled me to get in-depth knowledge in this subject. I took it as an online course, teachers are very knowledgeable and friendly. The course material designed by Dr Sonia is very valuable and easy to follow with all technical aspects. Cosmetology as a topic is covered very well in the manual. I also liked the practical sessions in their Mumbai center which provided me lot of training to use various equipments.

All the staff member at the center are friendly and I recommend to those who are aspiring to make a career in cosmetology to try this course.

As a Singapore Citizen I can assure that this course, its module and teaching is far more better than similar courses in Singapore. I am eager to join few more courses. Thank You once again.

—Ms Shreedevi Dileep, Singapore

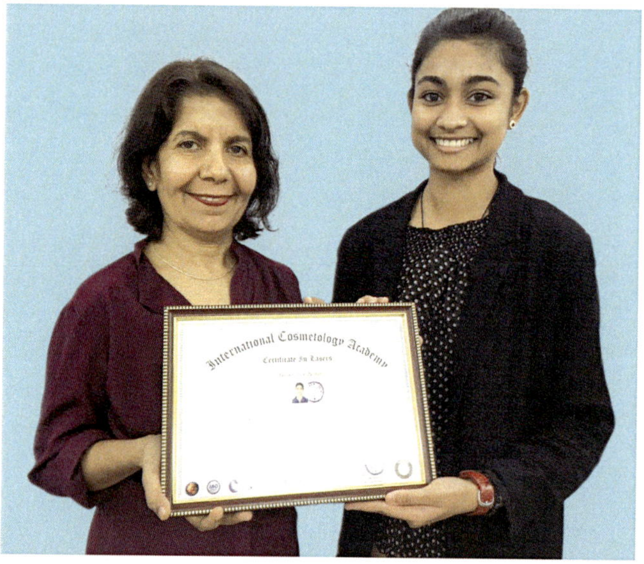

I came to know about Tender Skin Clinic through a family friend. My journey has been very good. The staff here is very helpful. I have got to learn new things after coming over here. Earlier I used to think that this field deals with beautifying a person artificially, but after doing the course I have understood that it deals with beautifying the skin scientifically. It was a very good and different experience to come to Tender Skin for all the courses which they provide.

—Ms Princhan Pulliwar, Dubai

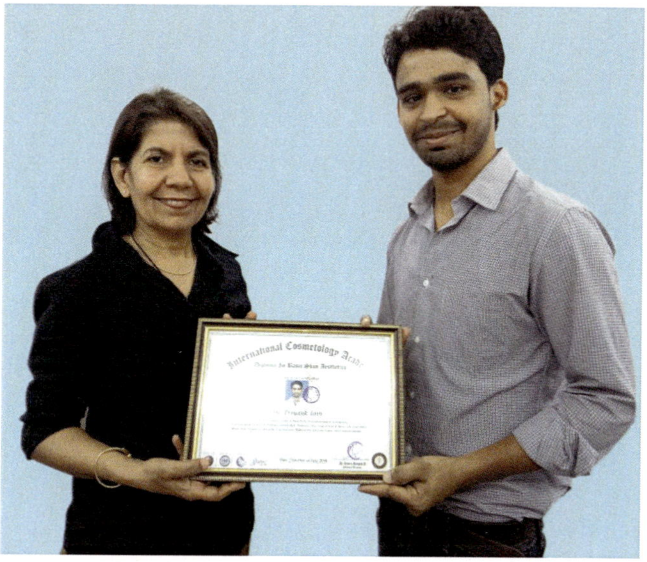

I had joined for all 3 levels—Diploma in Basic Skin Aesthetics, Diploma in Medical Skin Aesthetics and Certificate in lasers. It was very good experience doing the hands-on practice as I want to open my own center. After doing the procedures at the center, I felt more confident. I would like to thank Tender Skin to bring out the best in me.

—Dr Priyank Jain, Bhopal

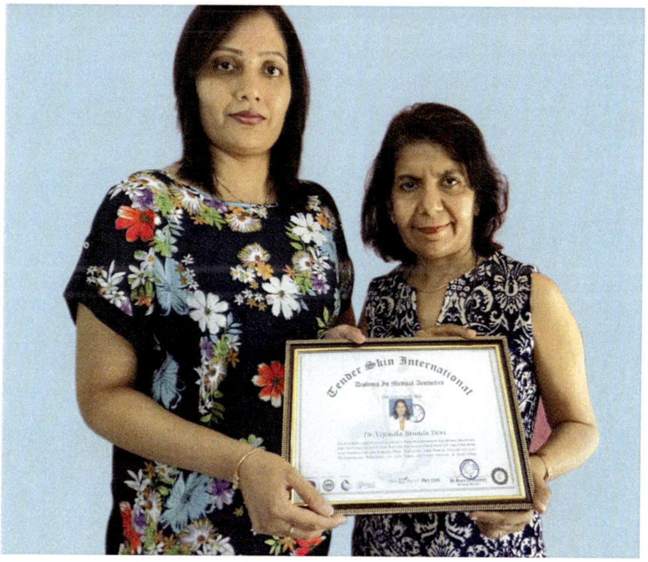

I searched on internet about cosmetology and I found Tender Skin International online. I researched about many other institutes but ultimately I joined Tender Skin International only. I joined on trial and error basis but after joining the course, the course curriculum was well structured so I selected this place but after joining this place I really liked this place, the course, the way they teach and about practical I must mention, they give more of hands-on practice. As there is a lot of growth I surely would suggest to select this course.

—Dr Brunda, Hyderabad

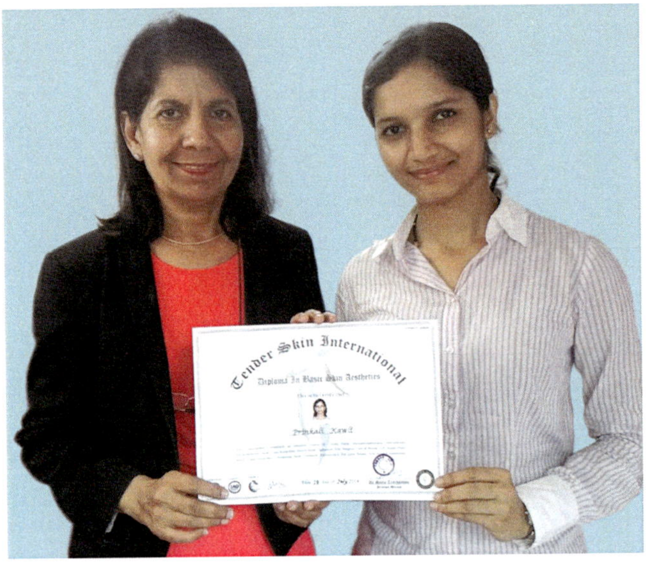

I have studied full cosmetology from this center. In the beginning I knew nothing, but after doing the course I realized there was lot to learn. After I was done with my course I got appointed and started working confidently. Thank you.

—Dr Prinkali, Boisar

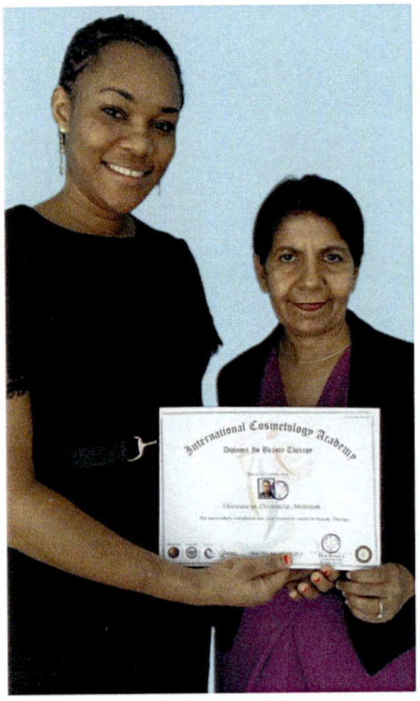

I come from Nigeria to study Beauty Therapy and going to Tender Skin International has been a pleasure to me. They have given me the exactly kind of knowledge that I need to know to move forward in the field of beauty and body care. I thank Dr Sonia for educating me in this field. I like all the treatments that I learned but my favorite has been radiofrequency and Peel for our every day maintenance of the skin. It has been a wonderful experience at the center.

—Ms Oluwaseyi, Nigeria

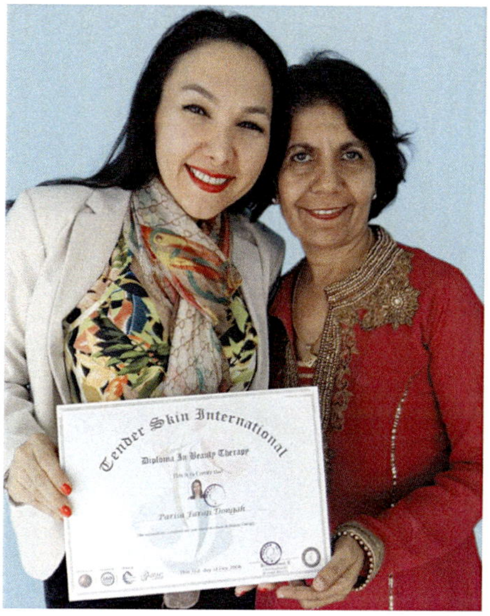

I have done my beauty course from Dr Sonia. It was a very good course, I learned a lot from her. I love her, her personality, the way she teaches, she is an amazing person. I highly recommend her to all the students who are looking out for the course in UAE. Thank you once again TSI for all the help.

—Ms Parisa, Tehran

Index

Page numbers followed by *f* refer to figure, *t* refer to table